Arthritis

An American Yoga Association
Wellness Guide

Arthritis

An American Yoga Association Wellness Guide

The Powerful Program for
Greater Strength, Flexibility, and Freedom

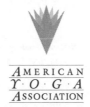

AMERICAN
Y·O·G·A
ASSOCIATION

Alice Christensen

The American Yoga Association

TWIN STREAMS
KENSINGTON PUBLISHING CORP.
http://www.kensingtonbooks.com

TWIN STREAMS BOOKS are published by

Kensington Publishing Corp.
850 Third Avenue
New York, NY 10022

ISBN 1-57566-648-0

Kensington and the K logo Reg. U.S. Pat. & TM Off.
Twin Streams and the TS logo are trademarks of Kensington Publishing Corp.

First Twin Streams Paperback Printing: March 2001
10 9 8 7 6 5 4 3 2 1

Printed in the United States of America

Photographs by Evelyn England, SAGE Productions
Hair and makeup by Estee Navarro and Ashley Kingston
Book design by Melody Oakes

READERS PLEASE NOTE: *The techniques and suggestions presented in this book are not intended to substitute for proper medical advice. Consult your physician before beginning any new exercise program. The American Yoga Association assumes no responsibility for injuries suffered while practicing these techniques. The American Yoga Association does not recommend Yoga exercise for pregnant or nursing women or for children under 16 years of age. If you are elderly or have any chronic or recurring conditions such as high blood pressure, neck or back pain, arthritis, heart disease, and so on, seek your physician's advice before practicing.*

Acknowledgments

I would like to thank the staff, students, and friends of the American Yoga Association for their help with this book, particularly Pattie Cerar and Carol Goodwin for general research assistance, Linda Gajevski for development and production, Stephen Grant for nutritional research and writing, and Patricia Rockwood for editorial assistance.

I would also like to thank the models for this book, including Steven Sanchez and Rodney Thompson, plus several students who have been with me for over 20 years: Patrick Benz, Pattie Cerar, Kent England, Artie Guerin, Carole Guerin, Anne Wardwell, and Ed Wardwell.

Table of Contents

Preface

I was diagnosed with rheumatoid arthritis in my late twenties. It was a devastating discovery. I had always been an active person, and the idea of slowly becoming debilitated by pain and deformity was unwelcome, to say the least. Rheumatoid arthritis was, and still is, considered a chronic disease from which one can find occasional relief, but not a cure.

I have learned that arthritis often shows in the body after a severe emotional upset or heavy stress. This certainly was true in my case. Rheumatoid arthritis bloomed suddenly in me after the loss of a baby girl. I just couldn't seem to recover, and as the months went on, my hands became swollen and extremely painful. As an attack came on, I would start to feel faint, and would gradually become unable to walk. I tried all kinds of pills to help the pain, especially aspirin, but with no relief.

I did not realize until much later that rheumatoid arthritis is sometimes related to an allergy — in my case, to coal tar, the substance used in most artificial colors and flavors. At the time, I didn't recognize it as an allergic reaction, but eventually, when I noticed that the progression of symptoms was always the same, I suspected allergy. I would feel a panic strike my body, and then the next day the arthritic pain would begin. The fear reaction reverberated throughout my whole being. My body was smarter than I knew: It was trying to tell me that something was not agreeing with me. I was fortunate indeed to find a great deal of relief from the symptoms by eliminating the substance from my diet.

When I went to a local allergy clinic to be tested, at first the physician was stumped, because I tested negative to every one of the usual allergens. Then he suggested coal tar, as he had read about its ability to cause allergic reactions. Unfortunately, a test for that allergy had not yet been developed. The doctor told me that in order to see if coal tar was indeed the problem, I would have to strictly eliminate it from my diet for an entire year.

I was in such pain that I decided to try what seemed to be impossible, and I embarked on the year's test. It was not easy. Any food or drink that contained artificial color or flavor had to be eliminated. This took hours of reading labels and adjusting my diet with foods that I could eat safely. My family was happy to go along with anything that would make me well. Vegetables and fruits became a big part of our menu. Very few processed foods met the requirements. We had to cut out all commercially made ice cream, as well as most bakery products and candy. Soft drinks, "junk food," chewing gum — all had to be carefully inspected. Even toothpaste was suspect. I made our ice cream in a hand-cranked churn; I also made all of our bread and other baked goods unless one of us discovered a coal-tar-free label. When that happened, it was welcomed as a great discovery, and we brought the booty home with the triumphant attitude of the "hunter home from the hill"!

Though I started my coal-tar odyssey in order to find some relief for my arthritis, it turned into a helpful exercise for my entire family. We all learned a lot. The food we ate was delicious, and we bloomed with health. By the time the year was up, my arthritis symptoms had subsided a great deal, so that I suffered only occasional flare-ups. I was deep into my study of Yoga by this time, and I believe that my practice of Yoga gave me the courage and insight to do something about my arthritis pain rather than simply suffer with it.

Pain is the central motivating force in dealing with arthritis. In my case, as I began my year of eliminating coal tar from my diet, it was a shock to realize that I could no longer take aspirin, because it was made with coal tar. I was not sure I could last a whole year without it, and I discovered a real fear reaction in myself at the idea of giving up what had helped relieve my pain. Fortunately, I learned that I didn't have to do without that help. I worked with a sympathetic doctor who was able to find pain-killers that had no allergenic substances in them.

I had to draw on all my reserves of courage. I was afraid to take too much medication for fear of addiction, and yet the severe pain sometimes left me no other avenue for relief. As I slowly built up my courage and strength by relying on my inner being, I realized that I was on my way to recognizing the power to change that was already a part of me, and that helped me to make the right choices. Yoga techniques helped me to strengthen myself from within.

I feel very fortunate to be able to tell you that I am no longer troubled with rheumatoid arthritis. After years of Yoga practice and careful monitoring of my diet, the attacks lessened. I slowly became more confident, and in 1963 I felt able to accompany my teacher Rama to India for advanced training in Yoga. We headed for his compound in the jungle above the town of Haridwar, where, for several months, I practiced silence and other techniques needed for my education in Yoga.

Suddenly, one day, a severe rheumatoid attack hit me in the hands and arms. You will smile when I tell you what Rama did:

He combined turmeric, onions, garlic, the leaves of the neem tree and various other plants, and flour, fried it all up in mustard oil and lathered it on my poor limbs where it hardened into a sort of cast, which I kept on for a couple of days. When the cast was broken, my hands and arms had returned to normal. I am happy to say they are still that way today and I haven't suffered any recurrence of pain or any other symptom.

I realize, of course, that not everyone heads for seclusion in the jungle and is fortunate enough to benefit from the priceless efforts of a great teacher to heal their woes. I am telling this story just to point out that sometimes we don't know what to do about arthritis. It is a mystery, and the real cause is not known. Every once in a while, however, help comes, sometimes from very unlikely sources. I hope you, too, will find help in your practice of Yoga. It has helped me to come through the siege of arthritis in my life with new strength and courage.

Long years ago, Rama told me, "Yoga makes the rough road smooth." This simple statement made a tremendous impression on me then, and it is a part of my constant remembrance today. I have learned that by applying the ethics and standards of the practice of Yoga in all the victories and defeats of my everyday life, I can achieve balance within myself, and the most difficult things become possible.

If you are in the battleground of constant struggle against the effects of arthritis, this book can help you gain the balance and confidence to live a full, productive life. I hope the contents will help you to heal and renew your body, supplying energy for movement and grace.

Alice Christensen

Introduction

The word "arthritis" means inflammation of the joints. Most people use the term to mean any painful condition of the joints, bones, or muscles, including bursitis, rheumatism, gout, and tendonitis, among many others. Arthritis affects people of all ages, although people over 50 are more likely to have osteoarthritis. Rheumatoid arthritis commonly afflicts younger people, primarily women. Rheumatoid arthritis is a severe inflammation that can affect other organs and tissues in the body besides the joints.

Arthritis can be caused by such varied factors as heredity, a malfunctioning immune system, the natural wear and tear of joints over time, infections, environmental reactions, injuries, and even allergic reactions to certain foods. Chronic anxiety and stress from personal problems can often cause a flare-up of arthritic symptoms.

The stress of chronic pain is probably the most prevalent feature of arthritis. Chronic pain affects all aspects of life. It often creates a cycle that begins with less and less physical activity, which results in discouragement, depression, and more inactivity. You feel trapped by your pain. You can't rest, you feel irritable, you are not up to dealing with other people, you have difficulty becoming interested in or concentrating on anything except the pain, and you may develop a greater dependence on narcotics, alcohol, or other drugs.

The brain naturally produces hormonelike chemicals, called endorphins, that closely resemble morphine. Endorphins are part of a natural pain-control system, and they are released as part of the brain's reaction to stress — but the supply is limited. Chronic stress, as experienced by those with chronic pain, may simply overwhelm the brain's ability to manufacture sufficient endorphins, leaving the individual more vulnerable to the ravages of stress.

Pain fosters inactivity, and it is important to remember that being inactive is usually the worst thing you can do for arthritis. Most physicians recommend a multidisciplinary approach to chronic pain that employs several methods for relief, including relaxation, gentle exercise, breathing, attention to diet, and guided imagery techniques — all of which may be found in the program in this book. Moderate exercise allows you to maintain optimum range-of-motion of your joints, and good nutrition makes sure that your body obtains the nutrients it needs to repair tissue, fight inflammation, and resist allergic reactions. A good diet will also help you lose weight if needed; even a little excess weight can sometimes make arthritis symptoms worse.

The program outlined in this book will be most successful for those of you who have mild to moderately severe symptoms of arthritis. Hundreds of people with varying types and degrees of arthritis have followed this program successfully over the years; however, everyone is different, and you may need to modify the program beyond the suggestions included in this book. I strongly suggest that you take this book to your personal physician and go over it together to make sure you are getting the most out of the program. This book cannot substitute for an ongoing relationship with the physician who is monitoring your arthritis, and you should never change your prescribed medication or regimen without consulting him or her.

Your Two Bodies

Successful change in the physical body calls upon the support of the inner emotional/spiritual body; change is never possible without a balance between the two parts. The idea that human beings have two bodies — the outer visible physical body that has a form, and the inner emotional/spiritual body that is formless — is central to all Yoga philosophy. The practice of Yoga is the process of bringing the two bodies together in balance. In other words, you develop a harmonious relationship with yourself.

Play a game with me. Stand in front of a mirror and look quietly at your whole reflection. Imagine your body as the outward picture of your personality. Does it really display the real you — the "you" that you wish to use as your vehicle in this world? I am willing to bet that you will find fault with your reflection, thinking such thoughts as, "I may look like this, but actually I am really someone else — someone inside me that doesn't show on the outside." This split usually causes the inner being, the unseen side of you, to take the outer, physical side of yourself to task. Usually, you will notice an uncomfortable, uneasy feeling in yourself, which has the effect of eroding your personal confidence.

Yoga philosophy describes this as "an awareness of separateness." This then becomes the central focus of our life, when we try to find balance, compassion, and oneness with both our bodies: the inner emotional/spiritual body and the outer physical body. Yoga techniques help to transform the battlefield between the two parts of ourselves into a peaceful ground of understanding and appreciation of the needs of both of the bodies that make up our whole existence. When dealing with the pain and crippling aspect of arthritis felt by your physical body, it helps to realize that you can call on your inner emotional body for support.

Most of us deal mainly with our physical body, although a few minor statements may be thrown like a bone to our inner body, such as "You made it to the bathroom without too much pain" or "This exercise routine is not as terrible as you thought it would be." Such placating statements imply that the inner body's force can be harnessed to the wants of the outer physical body's desires for change; it is supposed to "buckle down" and behave, and that's that!

But this is not what happens. The inner emotional body simply laughs and plays with us like an elephant with a mouse. It lets us have our egotistical game, and for a while the outer physical part of ourselves seems to control the show. We decide, "This body is mine and I am going to control it," and we go at it without asking for the cooperation of both bodies. In the end, the emotional body comes forward with force, demanding equal attention.

If the meeting of the two bodies does not take place, all efforts are bound to fail. The diet and exercise go on for a little while, but after some time the inner body tires of the game and comes back full force to return the outer physical body to its previous state, exactly as it was, very much like a fussy housekeeper who, every time someone moves a piece of furniture, hastily returns it to exactly the right position for her personal satisfaction. It seems paradoxical that a part of you would wish to return to a state of pain or discomfort, yet we often resist change because it represents the unknown, while staying as we are, even if it means being in pain, is familiar and seems less stressful. This becomes more and more true the longer the painful condition persists.

Successful management of arthritis can take place happily only when the two bodies are brought together in balance. If you truly want to change the way you feel, you must call a board meeting with yourself where both bodies are in attendance. Both bodies must be consulted for a happy agreement to the change.

It may be a difficult meeting at first, because the two bodies are not used to talking with each other, and this is not a meeting of equals! In fact, one has to wonder how the physical body ever got to the table at all. The emotional body is where your true strength lies; it is like a big cat disdainfully observing a nervous squirrel or a rabbit. The physical body has no idea of the power of the emotional body; it marches in demanding change as if it had all the answers. The emotional body listens and observes the physical's whining demands with lofty detachment. Each side maintains its separateness while the meeting goes on, and so nothing comes to agreement.

Try to imagine this scene played over and over again a hundred times as we try to change our lives. How many times have you tried to force your physical self to do something and failed? When the demands of the physical are put first, the body always suffers. I have observed people doing terrible things to their bodies in order to force a result. The emotional/spiritual body usually resents it so much that after a while it takes drugs, alcohol, or other destructive escapes to mask the upset.

Yoga philosophy believes that complete power lies in the inner body, the emotional/spiritual body, which never changes or dies. The fragile physical body, which is born and dies, actually only functions because of the strength and compassion of the inner body. If the two bodies can be encouraged to work together, the balance that is achieved makes any change possible.

This is the great contribution of Yoga techniques. The whole system of Yoga was designed exactly for this purpose. The word "Yoga" is a Sanskrit word that means "to join" or "to bridge." Yoga is used to bring both parts of yourself together to work in harmony. When this happens, the inner battles with yourself, that seem to be your constant companions, transform into clear bright insights of intuition and practicality. The expressions of the inner body's presence and power then are able to show in all the activities of your life.

Yoga practice shows you how to make the board meeting between your two bodies a success. If you give the unseen inner body expression, it will stop all resistance. It wants expression, and that can be done happily only if the outer physical body welcomes it. This friendly attitude developing in yourself then allows the strength of both bodies to come together in force, supporting all you want to do.

This book can teach you how to balance yourself so that, while you are changing, the fear of loss felt in both parts of yourself can be replaced with constant comforting and feeding while the changes are taking place — very much the way a child is raised to maturity when conditions are the most ideal.

Yoga offers a way to balance the expression of both bodies. Both will feel satisfied and be able to work happily together. Achieving this would mean that you become happy with the way you are. Those fortunate individuals who are happy with the way they are look beautiful. They shine with beauty from within that permeates their existence in the world. True, the exact perfection of the face and figure is usually not evident, and perfect health is hardly ever there, but it is not missed, because the beauty of the whole person displays itself, and we are enchanted.

Overview of This Book

I would like this book to give you a new way to approach arthritis, by learning how to move, breathe, eat, think, and feel, supplying proper attention to both your bodies.

Sometimes it helps to educate yourself about the situation you are facing. Chapter 1 outlines some basic information about arthritis. Chapter 2 provides a full description of our Yoga program, including a detailed discussion of how the various components of the program — exercise, breathing techniques, meditation, fantasy, moderate exercise, and diet — work together to help you reach your goals.

Our Yoga program for arthritis begins in Chapter 3, with complete instructions for the Yoga exercises, called asans, that I feel will be most helpful to you. We begin with a full range-of-motion sequence that also serves as a warm-up to the full Yoga exercise routine. Along with the exercise descriptions, I have included some additional material about the effects and benefits of each technique and some links to important nutritional advice. The program continues in the next three chapters: Chapter 4, with complete instruction in breathing techniques; Chapter 5, which teaches you how to relax completely and to meditate; and Chapter 6, which shows you how to use Fantasy to enhance your success. This chapter teaches one of my favorite exercises: the "I Love You" Meditation Technique. This is a wonderfully effective technique that many of my students have used with great success to help them feel better about themselves. In Chapter 7, I introduce a way to incorporate moderate activity using walking, swimming, or stationary cycling in your Yoga program in order to help you stay active.

Attention to diet and nutrition are essential components of wellness. A proper diet can improve your body's disease-fighting ability, repair tissues, and help you lose weight. Chapter 8 shows you how to modify your attitudes and tastes so that you can enjoy a healthy diet, with special attention to the components of your diet that will help you the most with arthritis. Chapter 9 discusses in detail the pros and cons of some of the most common alternative therapies that are being used today by arthritis sufferers. It contains specific recommendations that you can use to assemble your own trial program to assess its effectiveness for you.

The Resources section offers lists of support groups and organizations devoted to arthritis, helpful Internet sites, and a reading list on exercise and nutrition. This section also discusses how to choose a qualified Yoga teacher and presents a complete list of the American Yoga Association's books and tapes on Yoga for further study.

Cautions and Hints

Consult Your Physician

I advise all my new students to consult their physicians before beginning Yoga practice. Although the exercises and techniques in this book are meant for beginners, and are presented in a way that makes them easy to learn, it is a good idea to make sure that you have no underlying health problem that could cause complications. Your doctor can best tell you what movements you may need to avoid or modify in order to minimize your risk.

It is easy to modify the exercises in the routine if you are severely crippled due to arthritis or overweight. For many techniques, I've provided instructions for a seated version; you can easily adapt most of the other techniques the same way. If you have any questions about modifying the exercises in this book, please write to me at the address printed in the Resources section. My book *Easy Does It Yoga* is an excellent supplemental resource, as it provides dozens of adapted Yoga exercises that can be done in a chair, bed, or pool.

Set Realistic Goals

Do not strain to do more than your body can do happily; this would violate the important Yogic ethic of Nonviolence, and if your body is feeling pain, you won't enjoy your practices. If you try to do too much at first, it may soon feel overwhelming. I would like you to enjoy Yoga practice, not look upon it as pain or drudgery.

Very few people have the time or desire to do a full Yogic exercise program every day, and so I suggest starting with at least three of the exercises (in addition to the warm-ups) as your daily routine. Add more exercises whenever you wish, and gradually you will work into a fuller routine. I do suggest that you practice the warm-up exercises (pages 53-79) at least once a day — preferably twice or three times — because they provide full range-of-motion exercise for your joints, and it is important to work on that flexibility every day. Many of these can be done while watching television, for example.

I would like to stress that your total daily commitment to Yoga practice, including exercise, breathing, and meditation, should not take more than one hour; the ideal time for beginners is 20 to 30 minutes per day. Yoga seems very easy to do; however, it creates a powerful effect that is not always apparent when you are first starting out, and practicing for over an hour might upset your nervous system. You can practice in one continuous session or break your practice time into two 15-minute segments, morning and evening.

Many times, while talking to people I meet all over the world, I am dismayed to hear them say, "We do three hours of meditation every day," or "We always start with an hour of breath exercises." When I hear statements such as these, I have to suspect that the instructor is incompetent, because this intensity of practice is very hard on the nervous system. If students can truly meditate 10 to 15 minutes, that puts them at the top of my class. It takes many years to slip into long meditation, and it can never be forced. I suggest that you keep your daily routine short and interesting.

When to Practice

It does not matter what time of day you practice Yoga, although many people prefer early morning because their minds are not yet whirling with the day's activities. However, if you find that your joints are too painful in the morning, practicing in the evening is fine. Whatever time of day you choose, the most important thing to remember is to practice a little every day. Even if you practice only three exercises, three Complete Breath techniques, and a few minutes of meditation, you will continue to build an underlying momentum of regular Yoga practice that will eventually make it as easy and natural to do as brushing your teeth every day. You will miss it if you don't do it, because you find that both bodies are enjoying it.

Clothing, Equipment, Environment

Wear loose, comfortable clothing for Yoga practice, appropriate for the season. Try to keep these clothes separate so you use them only for Yoga practice. Do not allow yourself to become either chilled or overheated. It's best to practice Yoga exercises barefoot, but be sure to put on a pair of socks before you lie down for meditation in order to keep your feet warm. Also, wrap your upper body in a shawl or sweater when you meditate, because your body temperature will drop, and a chill can upset your meditation period.

You do not need any special equipment to practice Yoga other than a large towel, blanket, or mat that you use only for Yoga practice, and one or two small, firm cushions for the seated breathing exercises, if you wish to sit on the floor for these techniques. Alternatively, any sturdy chair that won't tip over will suffice. You can also practice most breathing techniques, and many of the Yoga exercises, lying in bed.

Choose a place in your home that is quiet and free from drafts. If you have small children at home, try to fit your practice into the times when they are asleep or at school, so that your attention is not split from what you are doing. Turn the volume on all your telephone equipment off so you will not be startled by loud noise, and be sure you will not be disturbed by pets.

Scheduling

Although the different parts of your Yoga routine — exercise, breathing, and meditation — will work best if done consecutively, sometimes your schedule or family obligations may not allow that much time all at once. In that case, it's fine to split up your routine. For instance, you could practice breathing and meditation in the morning and your exercise routine in the evening. Just be sure to practice a little every day without fail.

Food, Caffeine, Alcohol, Medication

Wait about two hours after eating a large meal so that you are not practicing Yoga exercises on a full stomach. However, a light snack or beverage before exercising will not hurt. Try to avoid practicing immediately after ingesting caffeine, and never practice Yoga under the influence of alcohol or street drugs. If you are taking any prescription medications that make you drowsy, wait until the effects have lessened before starting your Yoga routine.

Women's Issues

Women should not practice Yoga exercises during the heavy days of their menstrual cycle. The pressure of Yoga exercises on the internal organs may disrupt the natural hormonal changes of the body. Use the extra time for meditation, or spend a little more time on your walking exercises (see Chapter 7).

If you are pregnant or nursing, we do not recommend that you practice all the Yoga exercises because the changes in your body caused by the compression on internal organs may affect your child. A special routine for pregnant and nursing mothers is provided in two of our beginning books (see Resources). However, we do suggest that you continue your Complete Breath and meditation practice every day, as well as the Walking Contemplation exercise outlined in Chapter 7.

Supplemental Instruction

Yoga is best practiced alone, and I have designed this book to be your personal Yoga teacher. If you decide that you would prefer to supplement the course of study in this book with support from a local Yoga class, see the Resources for a discussion of some qualities to look for in a good Yoga teacher and a few suggestions about where to start looking. Also see the Resources for our excellent videotape that leads you through a basic 30-minute Yoga class such as I teach for the American Yoga Association.

I hope that you enjoy this program of Yoga for Arthritis. If you have any questions about what you are doing, please feel free to write to me at the address given in the Resources.

Chapter 1

Some Facts About Arthritis

Arthritis is the most prevalent, most often complained about condition in the United States. Surveys have indicated that as many as a third of all adults in this country have signs of arthritis such as swelling, pain, or limited motion. At any given time, about one in ten adults are experiencing neck pain, and the same proportion have had extended bouts with knee pain. The prevalence of arthritis is increasing and is expected to rise sharply for the next 20 years, as the population ages, to about 55 million people.

All forms of arthritis increase with age: About 5% of 18- to 44-year-olds have the disease, as compared with 28% of those aged 45 to 64, 46% of the 65 to 74 age group, and 51% of those 75 and over. Thus, the majority of the elderly have arthritis symptoms. Middle-aged and older people have more impairment from these diseases than from diseases in any other category. The disease is also biased according to gender: older women are about twice as likely as men to have some form of rheumatic disease. Of all the chronic conditions, arthritis and rheumatism account for more days lost from work and days spent in bed at home or with similarly restricted activities.

The term arthritis covers a host of conditions often unrelated to each other that affect all parts of the body. More than 100 different forms of arthritis are currently recognized. The most common conditions are osteoarthritis (affecting joint cartilage), bursitis (inflammation of the bursa, a sacklike tissue surrounding a joint), tendonitis (inflammation of a muscle-to-bone tendon), and low back pain. Bursitis and tendonitis are localized inflammations that usually appear and disappear suddenly, often within a matter of days or a few weeks. Less common forms of arthritis are rheumatoid arthritis (inflammation of the tissues surrounding joints), fibromyalgia (pain and tenderness in nonjoint tissue, along with a constellation of other symptoms such as sleep disturbance), and gout (crystal-induced joint inflammation).

Do You Have Arthritis?

The warning signs of arthritis are simply pain, swelling, stiffness, or difficulty in moving one or more joints. Most experts agree that if you experience any of these symptoms for more than two weeks, you should check out the cause with your doctor immediately. Remember that although more older adults get arthritis, it is not only an older person's disease; it can start at any age, even in childhood.

This book will be most helpful to you if you have mild to moderate osteoarthritis or rheumatoid arthritis. Many of the principles of our program may also be applied to bursitis and tendonitis. Fibromyalgia, gout, and low back pain are each so distinct that they cannot be effectively treated in this book. The same is true for systemic diseases that are related to arthritis, such as lupus, and various musculoskeletal conditions such as neck or shoulder pain, carpal tunnel syndrome, and so on. This is not to say that Yoga cannot be of benefit to you if you have these conditions; many of my students with fibromyalgia and other arthritislike conditions have found some relief from many symptoms with regular Yoga practice. Since everyone's experience of arthritis is different, I strongly suggest that you take this book to your doctor in order to be sure that you are doing what is best for your particular condition.

A Success Story

Recently we received this encouraging e-mail from Barb P. in Illinois:

"I have been having a really tough year beginning with a severely sprained ankle, that led to horrendous back pain after six months, that led to bursitis of the hip after all the exercise I did to get my back in shape again. I am 32 and felt like 100! My orthopedic surgeon suggested Yoga. I bought a Yoga video and started to do the routine as best I could, and my whole body seems like it is coming back to where it all should be. I am so happy that I am feeling better, and I really believe it is correcting my whole alignment and strengthening my weaknesses. Every time I do it, it is a little easier than the last time, and I haven't had to take any ibuprofen for quite a while (I was up to 12 a day)."

The remainder of this chapter will discuss osteoarthritis and rheumatoid arthritis in more detail, and outline the most common treatment options.

Osteoarthritis

Wear and tear on the joints is not the same as osteoarthritis, because arthritis can strike at any age, but wear and tear needs age to work its joint damage. Osteoarthritis is not a "symmetrical" disease; in other words, it can affect the left knee but not the right, or one hand but not the other, and so on, even if both have been subjected to the same wear and tear. Arthritis is more related to pressure and load on the joint than to frictional wear, and it progresses steadily over time, often resulting in joint immobility and pain.

High Heels and Arthritis

A group of British and American doctors, noting that women get osteoarthritis of the knee twice as often as men, decided to see if wearing high-heeled shoes could be a cause. In their study, 20 women averaging 36 years old walked across a special platform, first barefoot and then wearing 2 1/2-inch heels. Special sensors and cameras recorded the movements of ankle and knee joints in order to measure the strain on these joints. Among their findings was that wearing high heels puts greater strain on the inner side of the knee (a common site for osteoarthritis) than when walking barefoot.

Arthritis can be caused by some inborn abnormality of a joint or by an injury; this type is called "secondary arthritis." If there is no obvious cause, it is termed "primary." These distinctions often meld, however; for instance, those who develop arthritis after knee surgery are more likely to develop more generalized osteoarthritis. It appears that primary factors (genetic, metabolic, or hormonal) change the physical make-up of the joint cartilage, increasing the risk of developing osteoarthritis, whereas secondary factors, such as injury or repetitive strain, determine where and when osteoarthritis actually occurs.

The predominant symptom of osteoarthritis is pain, which can be due to inflammation or increased fluid pressure in the joint capsule. Pain is usually specific to a particular area or joint, not generalized. It is seldom severe, but tends to have a nagging quality that ebbs and flows depending on exertion, stress, or even the weather. This may be one reason there are so many folk remedies for arthritis: Because the symptoms come and go according to no obvious pattern, it can seem that they are eased with whatever remedy is popular at the moment. I'll talk more later in this chapter about some of the treatments that have been validated by scientific testing.

Usually, especially for mild to moderate arthritis, bed rest relieves the pain, although, as I will discuss later, prolonged bed rest can actually be bad for you. Stiffness is common, too, especially after periods of inactivity. Perhaps it is more noticeable in the morning upon arising, or after sitting still for some time. Gradually the stiffness may become permanent. Swelling and deformity of the joints may follow, along with loss of function of the joint.

Typically, osteoarthritis progresses very slowly, taking years for the symptoms to develop. Sometimes it disappears for months on end, possibly because the joint tissues are being repaired or restabilized by innate healing processes — although the body's capacity for this process tends to diminish somewhat with age. Many professionals fail to recognize this innate ability of the body to reshape or restabilize a damaged joint, sometimes quickly calling for intensive drug treatments or surgery without first trying less invasive methods to help the body heal itself.

The joints most often affected are in the hands, neck, lower back, hips, and knees. Ankles, wrists, elbows, and shoulders are only rarely involved. The symptoms — pain, tenderness, and swelling, along with limited movement — are typically experienced when doing everyday activities such as climbing stairs or using the hands. As osteoarthritis worsens, it takes less and less activity to cause joint pain.

Arthritis and Evolution

A novel theory has been proposed to account for the fact that hands, feet, knees, and hips are more commonly affected by arthritis than are ankles. Our joints developed in an evolutionary sense in the apes who used their arms extensively to help support their body weight. As humans evolved from apes and assumed an upright posture, the weight-bearing joints in the knees and hips were unable to cope with the greater stress. And as we humans developed our famous pincer grip, our hands also became vulnerable to cartilage damage. The theory also accounts for the increase of osteoarthritis with age, because the longer our incompletely adapted joints are exposed to excess joint stress, the more vulnerable our cartilage becomes to breaking down.

Osteoarthritis is also known as degenerative joint disease, because the cartilage, which cushions the ends of bones, breaks down. The function of cartilage is to lubricate the joints so that they move smoothly without friction. When cartilage does break down, the result is pain, swelling, and increasing stiffness. Although cartilage damage is still the principal cause of osteoarthritis, new evidence shows that in many cases the whole joint is involved: bones, soft tissue, joint membranes — even nearby muscles.

In a few cases, something other than accumulated joint stress can cause the loss of cartilage, such as a genetic problem in the joint, accidental injury, or inflammatory disease of some kind. Osteoarthritis itself is only rarely accompanied by inflammation, so it is a mistake to conclude that you have arthritis on the basis of common signs of inflammation, such as warmth or redness around the joint; instead, look for pain, stiffness, and lack of mobility as the first warning signs.

Who is Most at Risk for Osteoarthritis?

Not everyone will develop arthritis: overweight, joint injury, and genetics all play significant roles. Overweight is an important risk factor, especially for women, with the knee joint being most often affected. It seems obvious that the extra weight on the knees and hips leads to osteoarthritis by increasing pressure and load on the weight-bearing joints, but there is more to it than that, because even osteoarthritis in the hand increases with excess weight. For men and women both, shedding extra pounds is the most important thing you can do for yourself to maintain mobility and reduce joint stress. Losing weight reduces other symptoms besides joint pain, such as stiffness. Even more important, if you haven't yet experienced full-blown arthritis, you can lower your odds of developing osteoarthritis by 50% if you lose weight now.

Athletes may have a higher risk of osteoarthritis, not because of repetitive wear and tear, but rather due to major joint injury, in the same way that an accident or other injury affecting a joint may lead to osteoarthritis in a nonathlete.

Those who work in occupations that require certain types of repetitive movements are more at risk. For example, jobs requiring heavy lifting with knee bending, or those requiring a fine finger grip, especially the "pincer" movement, such as writing with a pen or pencil for long periods of time, are associated with higher rates of osteoarthritis.

Treatments for Osteoarthritis

When I was growing up, cortisone was a relatively new discovery and was thought at first to be a "miracle cure" for arthritis, but physicians soon discovered that they did not know how to use it safely and effectively as a long-term treatment. Aspirin and gold injections were the only other treatments available.

Patient education, weight loss, exercise, and occupational therapy to find better ways to support painful joints and still take care of business are the main strategies that should be in place before trying more aggressive drug or surgical remedies. Educating yourself and your family about arthritis can be very beneficial. Contact a local chapter of the Arthritis Foundation for the Arthritis Self-Help course (see Resources). These programs are proven to help reduce pain and improve the overall quality of life.

New Treatments for Arthritis

Recently two dietary supplements have been shown to be beneficial for osteoarthritis: glucosamine and chondroitin sulfates. Both have been extensively tested and found to be both safe and effective, although most scientists feel that more research is needed to be sure of the extent of benefit as well as any cautions. Both substances have antiinflammatory effects, and both stimulate cartilage metabolism. These may be the only two compounds capable of actually modifying the affected joint. X-ray evidence has clearly shown favorable changes in many cases. One study of patients with arthritis in their knees who were treated with glucosamine over a three-year period showed that the progression of the disease had been halted. The reduction in symptoms by these substances is well established, although the size of the benefit is still to be determined. The National Institutes of Health have recently begun a large, definitive study involving 1,000 people with osteoarthritis. (For more about dietary supplements for arthritis, please see Chapter 9.)

If you have an impaired ability to walk, care for yourself, cook, shop, or perform your usual work or hobby satisfactorily, you may benefit greatly from consultation with physical and occupational therapists. These professionals can teach you how to improve your strength and flexibility and find new ways to perform activities that have become problematic.

Aerobic activities such as walking and swimming are usually helpful, leading to decreased pain, depression, and anxiety, and improved fitness. The Yoga program in this book includes a section on how to gradually add moderate exercise to your routine (see Chapter 7).

Pain relief is the first order of business when considering drug therapy, and acetaminophen (the main ingredient in Tylenol) is the preferred over-the-counter remedy. Acetaminophen toxicity is very rare; a few people who consume too much alcohol while taking the drug have liver problems. Also still widely used are the NSAIDs ("NonSteroid Anti-Inflammatory Drugs" such as aspirin and ibuprofen). Recently, however, professionals have become concerned about the harmful effects of the NSAIDs on cartilage; it appears that these drugs may actually make the condition for which they are prescribed even worse. NSAIDs also can have a harmful effect on the gut (see p. 31).

Although quite new, the COX-2 inhibitors (Celebrex and Vioxx, discussed in more detail on p. 32) are rapidly becoming the first prescription drug your physician will prescribe, often with a suggestion to supplement it with acetaminophen for extra pain relief. If these drugs are insufficient, then your physician will probably prescribe a stronger painkiller, possibly followed by other, more powerful NSAIDs. If all else fails, joint surgery or replacement is often the treatment of last resort.

For those with knee problems, strengthening of the thigh (quadriceps) muscle reduces pain and improves mobility. Fitness walking has also proven beneficial. Pain-relieving creams are helpful for joint pain. Later in this chapter, I will discuss various general therapies for arthritis in more detail.

Rheumatoid Arthritis

Rheumatoid arthritis affects more than two million Americans (about 1 per 100 adults). There is no known cause, cure, or means to prevent rheumatoid arthritis. The trick is to detect the condition early enough to prevent irreversible joint damage.

This is an autoimmune disease — meaning that the body's own immune system attacks the body's tissues — resulting in symptoms of redness, swelling, tenderness, and heat at affected joints. Rheumatoid arthritis is caused by the inflammation of the membrane lining a joint, and most joints in the body may be affected. During the inflammation, the body's own immune system invades the joint and can cause loss of bone and cartilage, leading to loss of mobility and pain. The joint actually loses its normal shape and alignment if the inflammation and autoimmune reaction are not treated. Rheumatoid arthritis is often preceded by flu-like symptoms lasting several weeks. Fatigue, fever, weakness, general pain, and stiffness usually appear before painful, swollen joints. This general feeling of illness and malaise emphasizes both the systemic nature of the disease (it affects the whole body) and also its autoimmune nature: the body reacts as if it were fighting an infection or other foreign substance.

The autoimmune reaction can be caused by a genetic susceptibility, though this is less common; most of those closely related to someone with the disease do not get it. More often, some type of environmental trigger, possibly a virus or bacterium, or a food or other allergen — as happened in my case — can be blamed. Rheumatoid arthritis occurs more frequently with age and is widespread among all races and around the world. It seems to be closely related to hormonal levels; it is more common in women, and often diminishes during pregnancy. Men with rheumatoid arthritis have low testosterone levels; women using oral contraceptives have lower rates of the disease. Low levels of vitamin E, beta-carotene, and selenium, powerful antioxidants in the blood, are associated with increased risk. Those most severely affected have a lifespan about ten years shorter than average; they die more often from infection, kidney disease, and intestinal bleeding than those without the disease.

Unlike osteoarthritis, rheumatoid arthritis usually is symmetrical, affecting both sides of the body more or less equally: both hands, for instance. If the disease progresses, bone and cartilage in the affected joints can erode, resulting in pain, impaired function, and disability. Impairment and disability result in limited physical activity in general, and loss of specific activities of daily living.

Today, if rheumatoid arthritis is detected at an early stage, damage to joints can be limited with a combination of drug treatment, exercise, and lifestyle modification. Yoga is in many ways

Laughter Medicine

Some rheumatoid arthritis sufferers have found at least temporary relief through laughter. Doctors say there's more to it than just taking your mind off the pain. The pain of rheumatoid arthritis is primarily caused by muscle spasm, and the muscle contraction and relaxation involved in laughter tends to override other muscle spasms, causing those other muscles to relax and feel less painful.

an ideal complement to your physician's prescribed treatment, offering a beneficial form of exercise, stress management skills, and positive dietary changes that powerfully augment traditional therapies. The Yoga program for arthritis is outlined in more detail in Chapter 2.

Rheumatoid arthritis can be very aggressive, rapidly eroding joint tissues and causing irreversible joint damage, so it is essential for your physician to regularly monitor the disease. Patient education, self-help rehabilitation activities, and initial treatment with NSAIDs may be sufficient to protect the joints. As with osteoarthritis, it is likely that the newer COX-2 inhibitors (see p. 32) will be prescribed by your physician in an attempt to control the inflammatory response and protect the joints. If these are insufficient, then more powerful NSAIDs, corticosteroids, hydroxychloroquine, gold therapy, penicillamine, azathioprine methotrexate, and cyclophosphamide are some of the drugs commonly used. If all else fails, then joint surgery or replacement may be called for.

Yoga and Rheumatoid Arthritis in Britain

Even those with severe rheumatoid arthritis can benefit from Yoga practice, according to a British trial. As compared with a control group, a group of patients following an intensive Yoga class for about three months experienced less disability and greater hand grip strength. The classes included classical Yoga poses, breathing techniques, meditation, Yoga philosophy, and techniques to "soften the emotions." Movements were modified to avoid strain when joints were inflamed.

Treatments for Arthritis

Arthritis does not necessarily win, and disability is not inevitable. If you are determined to help yourself, you need to commit a serious amount of time and energy. If you do, you will be rewarded with much less impairment and disability, and you can even control inflammation, if it is present. In fact, control of inflammation is the cornerstone to reducing or halting the progress of rheumatoid arthritis.

Since arthritis is chronic, you may experience feelings of frustration and even failure as you strive to continue your self-care program over the long haul. If you don't address those feelings, you could become depressed, and stop taking care of yourself, leading to a worsening of your condition. This is one of the ways Yoga practice can be so helpful to you. Our program includes many techniques that counter common feelings such as these and help you remain positive and energetic. As I mentioned in the Introduction, helping yourself involves more than just treating your physical body; your inner emotional body needs a great deal of attention, because this is where your true strength lies. There is a lot you can do to keep both your bodies balanced and healthy, so don't be discouraged.

Weight Loss

As I mentioned previously, the most important thing you can do for arthritis is shed extra pounds (or maintain your ideal weight). Overweight definitely increases the risk of arthritis, especially of the knee, and even more so for women.

Rest

Rest can help reduce the inflammation of rheumatoid arthritis; in fact, prolonged bed rest was often prescribed before much was known about the disease. Currently, however, professionals believe that a combination of short periods of rest and an appropriate exercise and training program are more beneficial, because bed rest can severely reduce mobility in a very short time. For example, bed rest may result in the loss of three percent of muscle strength in just one day; you can see how quickly that would add up to severe weakness if you remained in bed for several days.

If you need a few days' bed rest to deal with an acute flare-up of rheumatoid arthritis, then you can exercise in bed to prevent loss of muscle tone. (Many of the Yoga exercises in our program can be modified to be done in bed; see Chapter 3 for some ideas, or consult my book *Easy Does it Yoga*.) A better solution is to rest for a limited period each day, or just rest a particular joint. For instance, try one hour of bed rest during the day to combat the fatigue, and use braces to rest specific joints (for instance, a wrist splint).

Exercise

The natural response we all have to pain is to stop moving; for a short period of time, as I discussed above, rest can help reduce inflammation, especially in cases of rheumatoid arthritis. However, it's important to counteract that tendency to remain immobile for long periods, because you need to exercise to keep the range of motion of your joints at its best, to maintain muscle strength, and to reduce pain.

How Does Exercise Help to Reduce Pain?

Although it may seem contradictory, much of the pain of arthritis comes from inactivity, which stiffens the joints. Exercise keeps your joints mobile and helps your body to heal itself. Joints are encapsulated tissues that naturally and regularly tear down and rebuild, just like other tissues in your body; movement, which improves circulation, makes it easier for the joint to excrete waste products and bring in the building materials that it needs to support repair and rebuilding.

Exercise is the best way to increase your feeling of vitality, because it reduces fatigue and promotes a sense of well-being: You will look and feel better for every minute you exercise! If you have arthritis, perhaps you fear the consequences, such as loss of independence or your job, and social isolation. Many people fear becoming disabled, and suffer diminished self-esteem and depression as a result. Actively participating in your own rehabilitation with the program outlined in this book can be a powerful antidote for these common feelings.

Exercise, of course, is absolutely essential for maintaining your ideal weight. Exercise also helps increase strength and endurance, making it easier to stick to an exercise program as well as making it easier to perform everyday tasks. Exercise also helps to prevent loss of bone density, especially important for older women, who may already be losing bone density due to menopause.

Exercise also helps keep the joints from "freezing" in a particular position. Arthritic joints tend to feel most comfortable in a slightly flexed position, and without movement the joint may tighten in this position permanently. Even the surrounding muscles and tendons may shrink, adding to the loss of mobility and increasing pain. Exercise helps to increase range of motion, endurance, strength, and coordination throughout your body. For instance, exercising your hand may help maintain the strength of your grip and pinching movements, as well as strengthening your arm muscles. If you have osteoarthritis of the knee, exercise not only increases the mobility in your knee joint, but also strengthens your leg muscles, improving your ability to walk, climb stairs, drive, and do other common daily activities.

Yoga for More Limber Hands

A ten-week study involving Yoga classes for people with osteoarthritis of the hands resulted in less pain, less tenderness, and greater finger range of motion than a control group that followed a drug-based treatment program. Besides the classical Yoga techniques, the weekly classes included group discussions and lots of social support.

You can experience the benefits of exercise at any age; even the frail elderly can gain strength and mobility by starting to exercise regularly. Experts say there are three types of exercise you need: range of motion, strength, and endurance. Our Yoga program includes all three. Even if you start with only the range-of-motion exercises (see pp. 53-79) and do them once or twice daily, you will notice a quick improvement.

Sometimes applying heat to your affected joints and taking pain medications before you start your exercise session can increase the effectiveness and comfort level of exercise. Don't use heat therapy on acutely inflamed joints, and do not put too much stress on hips and knees by running or jogging when these joints are acutely inflamed. Low-impact aerobic exercise such as walking or swimming — such as the program outlined in Chapter 7 — is usually beneficial.

It is important to exercise at least 30 minutes daily; do your program at a time of day when pain and stiffness are less. During acute flare-ups of inflammation, just focus on maintaining range of motion (the warm-up exercises in Chapter 3). As a general guide, exercise every joint through its full range of motion at least three times, twice daily. When pain and stiffness abate, try to restore joint mobility, strength, and aerobic fitness by gradually adding more vigorous exercise a little at a time.

Support Groups

Although Classical Yoga suggests that best results are obtained by practicing alone, I suggest that you also work with an exercise group. Years of experience have demonstrated good results from structured group exercise classes for people who are following a self-help program for arthritis. A structured class will help you enormously to keep up a daily practice over the long term, it will provide good company, and it will not interfere with your Yoga program. Swimming and bicycling programs are also helpful. Contact your local Arthritis Foundation chapter for help in finding a group near you.

Medication

Currently, as I discussed previously, the first line of defense against arthritis is a class of drugs called NSAIDs, which has evolved to include everything from the lowly aspirin and the now common over-the-counter ibuprofens (Advil, Motrin) to Feldene, Voltaren, Nalfon, Indocin, Naprosyn, Tolectin, and Clinoril. All of them share aspirin's ability to block the body's production of prostaglandin, which is how the body actually produces inflammation. This shared feature has prompted the retranslation of the mnemonic NSAID to be "New Sorts of Aspirin In Disguise"! These drugs are commonly used to treat most, if not all, forms of arthritis and have been proven effective in reducing the swelling, tenderness, and pain of the disease.

However, the constant use of NSAIDs can have toxic side effects, especially for older people. One problem is a greater risk of peptic ulcer, with the associated risk of bleeding and perforation of the gut. This is a very serious problem: in the United States alone, approximately 60,000 hospital visits each year by arthritis patients are directly attributable to NSAID-induced gut problems. In addition, authorities estimate that 3,000 deaths each year are directly linked to NSAID effects. Approximately one person per hundred taking one of the NSAIDs daily for six months or longer will experience ulcers and complications. Additionally, the NSAIDs can cause ulcerative colitis in the colon.

You are at risk for GI tract bleeding caused by NSAIDs if you are age 65 or older, have a history of ulcers or upper GI bleeding, or use oral steroids (such as Cortisone) or anticoagulant drugs (such as Coumadin). Smoking and alcohol consumption also increase risk. If you are sensitive to aspirin, you need to take extra care.

Ironically, the same feature of NSAIDs that benefits arthritis sufferers by reducing inflammation — the blocking of prostaglandin production — is what increases the risk of gut problems. Normal prostaglandin production is necessary to protect the gut: it stimulates the stomach and duodenal blood flow as well as mucus and bicarbonate secretion. Without the protection of prostaglandins in the gut, the digestive enzymes and acids would literally "eat" right through the walls of the gut. This same prostaglandin production, however, is also responsible for the inflammation of the arthritic joints and soft tissue, with the associated pain, swelling, and other symptoms.

The search for drugs that reduce the inflammation of arthritis without blocking the protective action of gut prostaglandins has been the "Holy Grail" of pharmaceutical research. The "good" prostaglandin, or COX-1, molecule was identified in the mid-1970s, and in the early 1990s, the second form, COX-2, which is only produced at sites of inflammation (for example, an arthritic joint), was identified. The new drugs, therefore, had to inhibit the action of only COX-2, without blocking the gut-protection role of the COX-1 molecule.

Newer drugs are now available that markedly reduce the risk of GI tract complications: a class of drugs that have the benefit of aspirin's antiinflammatory action, but without the risk of ulcers. They are called COX-2 inhibitors, and two are currently approved: celecoxib (Celebrex) and rofecoxib (Vioxx). These newer prescription-only drugs appear to effectively reduce the risk of gut problems, especially ulcers, to normal levels. These drugs are prescribed to reduce the pain and stiffness of arthritis, which makes a big difference in increased mobility for therapeutic exercise as well as normal daily activities.

Heat and Cold

Cooling causes blood vessels to temporarily constrict, and heat has the opposite effect. No one really seems to know why or how heat helps with joint pain; its use goes back to ancient times in the form of mud baths, mineral waters, and hot springs. The heat or cold does not penetrate to deep joints and muscles; nonetheless, heat and cold application does reduce pain, enhance stretching, and relax tight muscles. Some suggest the best form of therapy is to alternate: first hot packs, then cold ones. A good general rule is to try cold therapy when inflammation is acute or when an injury is fresh (within the first 24 hours) and try moist heat therapy or alternating heat-and-cold therapy when pain and inflammation are mild and chronic.

Various means to provide heat and cold are available, ranging from hot water bottles and heating pads to gel packs that can be frozen or microwaved as needed. Always use caution, especially with electric pads, so be sure to follow the manufacturer's directions concerning use around water and falling asleep with one in place. Paraffin wax dips are particularly useful for hands as the wax molds itself to the contours of the joints and retains warmth for 20 minutes or so. When using cooling packs, be sure to protect the skin with a towel or other barrier to prevent direct contact with freezing temperatures.

Chapter 2

How Yoga Can Help Arthritis

The arthritis management program presented in this book is designed to help you cope with pain and stiffness, improve range of motion, lose weight if necessary, increase your strength for daily activities and overall disease resistance, and learn to see yourself not as a victim of arthritis but as a person for whom arthritis is a minor, occasional inconvenience. Our program teaches a lifestyle change: If you follow our guidelines, you will think differently, move differently, relax, breathe, and even eat differently. By making these techniques and ideas a part of your everyday life, you will have a much greater chance of maintaining your independence and reducing discomfort.

This is a six-part program based on traditional Yoga techniques. Among the techniques that you will learn in this book are physical exercises, breathing techniques, meditation training, fantasy exercises, attention to diet, awareness of ethics, and a special contemplation exercise to practice while doing moderate exercise. Here are some of the ways these techniques work:

• **EXERCISE.** The Yogic school of exercise, called asans, was developed for the body to maintain balanced mental and physical health. Yoga asans apply pressure to the glandular system of the body. This helps the body to stay strong and totally balanced. This glandular pressure also promotes the release of the chemicals, called endorphins, that cause feelings of well-being in the brain. This aspect of Yoga practice can be very helpful in relieving depression, anxiety, and insomnia. Yoga asans help to improve strength, flexibility, vitality, posture, and muscle tone, which will help you look and feel better, the idea being that the road to health lies in your own body. Yoga exercise contributes to a preventive system that helps avoid the vicious cycle of pain, leading to inactivity, leading to more pain.

• **BREATHING.** Yoga breathing techniques nourish your inner body by helping to reduce anxiety and depression and create calm, clear, and creative thinking. The ancient Yoga teachers describe a mysterious way that breathing techniques cleanse the nervous system, making its full function available for body needs. Breathing exercises also develop a depth of sensitivity which is very helpful in dealing with your inner emotional spiritual body. The effects are especially noticeable when you spend some extra time trying to begin a new relationship with yourself.

Many people first come to Yoga in order to reduce their stress responses. This is a wonderful "side effect" of practicing Yoga that will help you learn how to cope with the inevitable anxieties of life with arthritis, especially if you are undergoing the additional stresses of coping with pain or trying to lose weight. Many people report that concentrating on their breath helps reduce pain as it relaxes the body.

• **MEDITATION.** Yoga meditation techniques increase self-awareness and augment the balanced, calming effects of exercises and breathing techniques. In the practice of meditation, the physical body is quieted and all inner conversation is silenced for a short time. This allows the intuitive voice, which is the language of the inner emotional body, to speak. This intuitive voice is the gateway for expression that the inner spiritual body seeks, and it provides comfort from within. Meditation is one way to acknowledge your inner emotional body.

• **FANTASY.** Guided Yoga Fantasy techniques enhance self-esteem and counter the "victim" mindset felt by many sufferers of arthritis. Through practice of these techniques, which you can use throughout the day during many activities of daily life, you will learn that your inner thoughts and feelings determine your image of yourself and how you face and behave in the world. Regular practice of these Fantasy exercises will help you build and sustain a new image of yourself as you wish to be.

• **MODERATE EXERCISE.** Moderate-intensity exercise helps to burn calories, build muscle, and improve cardiovascular fitness. In our program, we teach you how to perform this moderate exercise at your own pace and with a Yogic mind of centered attention: a quiet meditative focus on your inner self. The best all-around moderate-intensity exercise is walking; it can be done by almost anyone, and it can be done safely while centering your attention on one of the contemplation exercises introduced in Chapter 7. Walking can be done outside in any safe environment, or inside on any suitable treadmill. Other forms of exercise that will work with this technique are swimming and riding a stationary bicycle.

• **DIET AND SUPPLEMENTATION.** An arthritis diet is essentially a well-balanced diet emphasizing whole foods and fresh fruits and vegetables. Many arthritis sufferers need to lose weight; Chapter 8 provides some tips for losing weight at a slow but steady rate. An important component of this section is recommendations for changing your taste preferences in foods to emphasize healthier choices while not giving up enjoyment. Because there are so many alternative diets and dietary supplements recommended for arthritis, we take a good hard look at the most popular and provide some recommendations in a separate chapter.

These are the basic components of our Yoga Program for Arthritis. Before starting to teach you the routine itself, I'd like to discuss the role of ethics in Yoga practice and arthritis, and introduce you to a wonderful motivational technique that has worked well for many of my students.

Ethics in Yoga

Many times, Yoga is misunderstood as religious. Yoga is not a religion; it is a way to find yourself, a joining, a bridge to the unknown parts of yourself. The science of Yoga provides tools that can be used by people of any faith or background to enhance their lives. Throughout this book, I've used the term "emotional/spiritual" to refer to your inner body; I do not use the word "spiritual" in a religious sense but rather as a way to indicate that something else within you, besides your familiar physical and mental processes, is also deeply involved in your health and well-being. This inner self is often unknown to us until we learn how to pay attention to it, and Yoga techniques are a way to welcome the participation of this inner being.

One of the most important aspects of Yoga is the practice of ethics. Yoga philosophy teaches that ethics are the gateway to the inner self. In other words, you can only fully experience the participation of your emotional/spiritual body with the help of an awareness and practice of ethical behavior. Yoga holds great reverence for life, and for this reason, the ethic of Nonviolence becomes its mainstay. This is especially important when trying to deal with pain. Many people adopt the attitude that pain can somehow be "good for you," that it "builds character," and that those who complain about it are weak. In the view of Yoga, the ethic of Nonviolence applies first and foremost to yourself.

A woman I know contracted rheumatoid arthritis several years ago in her early thirties. At first she consulted a nutritionist who put her on a strict diet — vegetarian, gluten-free, sugar-free — and she noticed a relief from symptoms in a few months. However, she did not stay on the diet because, as she told me, she felt that it was too restrictive, and she couldn't stand the thought of not being able to eat the things she liked for the rest of her life. Now she is back primarily to a traditional American diet that includes meat, alcohol, sugary foods, and other things that she knows contribute to the inflammation of rheumatoid arthritis, yet she seems to be willing to suffer in order to eat what she wants.

I believe that if you learn to connect to your inner emotional/spiritual body through the practice of ethics, particularly Nonviolence, you will not experience this type of conflict, because the longer you practice, the more you will become able to see your dietary changes and other techniques not as harsh disciplines but as enjoyable practices that will free you from pain and dependence. In one of the most well-known Yogic texts, the *Bhagavad Gita*, there is a phrase that explains this phenomenon perfectly. It says, in talking about establishing regular practice, that it seems "like poison in the beginning, but like nectar in the end." When you first begin your arthritis management routine with this book, it may seem like a lot of effort and may even be a little uncomfortable, especially if you are used to not moving at all in order to avoid pain. With practice, however, you will find that your Yoga routine becomes habitual and quite enjoyable as you gain strength and reduce your discomfort.

Many experts in the field of psychology have discussed the fact that humans have an innate tendency toward self-annihilation ("thanatos") that constantly battles with the body's natural instinct for survival ("eros"). You can see this in people who turn to drugs, alcohol, and other self-violent behaviors in an attempt to escape from pain or depression, not realizing that they are only making their condition worse.

Yoga philosophy recognizes these opposing forces and teaches students to be aware of both tendencies as they make choices in life. The study of ethics in Yoga is the best way to recognize when you are being violent toward yourself so that you can choose to behave differently. The *Gita* says, "You are your own best friend and your own worst enemy." By consciously choosing a healthy lifestyle while acknowledging the other choices that you have left behind, you will develop increasing strength that will carry you through anything that you do in life.

Regular daily practice of the Yoga program outlined in this book will prepare your physical body to join with your inner emotional body without pain or upset. The results show very quickly. You should feel the difference in just two or three days. It is hard to describe this change, because the body does not change quickly, but the feelings that accompany regular practice are so pleasant that you won't want to give it up; these feelings reflect the participation of your inner body in the healing process. The two bodies at the board meeting can finally talk to each other as the rift of separateness heals, giving you the full power to be what you want to be.

Those who take up the practice of Yoga in this nonviolent way rarely ever stop. Thousands of people who have always hated to exercise and have been unable to maintain a happy daily discipline now look forward to their daily practice of Yoga. You will never fear it; in fact, you will really miss your practices if you don't do them. You don't have to go to a class to achieve this effect; practicing at home alone with this book, or with a class videotape such as our *Basic Yoga* (see Resources), will give you wonderful results.

A regular daily routine of Yoga exercises, breathing, meditation, and fantasy, even if it lasts only a few minutes, will produce happy, comforting expression from the inner emotional body. When this happens, healing begins.

The Wrist Tape Technique

Now I am going to introduce you to a wonderful motivational tool that you can use to help you succeed in your arthritis management program. My students have great luck with this technique, which they use when they want to change something in their behavior. It is extremely successful in the practice of ethics or any other behavioral change that you wish to attempt.

Let's say you want to become more aware of how often during the day you do or say something that is hurtful to yourself. To try the Wrist Tape exercise, simply place a small piece of nonirritating tape, such as first aid-type adhesive tape, a Band-Aid, or painter's masking tape, on the inside of your wrist or on a watch band. Every time you notice yourself doing or saying something that is violent to yourself, make a mark on the tape. For instance, if you look in the mirror and think negatively about your appearance, that would be a violent thought; if you are trying to lose weight but you eat an extra dessert anyway, that would be a violent act. At the end of the day, paste the tape on your refrigerator door. By the week's end you will see a row of tapes indicating how you have progressed in acting on your new vision of yourself.

Using a Wrist Tape to Practice Nonviolence

Here is what one student wrote to me about her practice of this technique: "When I caught myself in a violent thought and made a mark, it was as if I was able to let it go, instead of grinding and grinding about whatever it was that was upsetting me. I know this connection is nebulous, but somehow it helped me to see that nothing is outside of myself; that all those things that I thought were out there upsetting me were actually reflections of my own self — my unconscious self that I tend to forget to talk to, even though I've been trying every day to take time out to give it voice. It's made me take another look at the way I've been trying to run my life."

This practice promotes great respect for yourself because it shows you the great effort you are putting into your lifestyle change. When you are able to perceive the effort clearly, you will be able to really congratulate your inner emotional spiritual body for its support in the process. This will begin to bring you together with your emotional self in a nonviolent process that will develop a friendly support within yourself for what you want to do.

Be Kind to Yourself

Now you are ready to begin our complete Yoga Arthritis Management Routine. Don't worry if you cannot do the complete routine all at once. In fact, if you have not exercised in a long time, it will be much more beneficial to start slowly, doing one or two exercises each day and adding techniques as you gain strength and stamina. Always try to practice a little every day, however. This daily consistency will give momentum to your efforts and result in quicker and longer lasting results.

Here is a suggested schedule for the first week, incorporating each of the six parts of our program, illustrating how to increase your practice gradually over several weeks:

Exercise

All warm-ups, plus three exercises (add one to two new exercises each week).

Breathing

Three Complete Breaths (add three repetitions each week until you reach one minute total; next try the

Sitali breath technique and build up to one minute over several weeks; finally add the Alternate Nostril Breath and the Bellows Breath and build up to one minute. Your total practice of breath techniques at one sitting will never exceed four minutes. Of course, you can practice breathing techniques at other times of the day as described in Chapter 4).

Meditation

Five minutes (add three minutes per week until you reach 20 minutes — about six weeks; stay at this length of time indefinitely, or continue to 30 minutes in three-minute intervals as before).

Fantasy

"Creating a Vision of Yourself." (Practice this every day for one week, then try a new Fantasy exercise the same way during the following week and the week after. Then alternate techniques as you wish, or practice them combined with your activity program as described in Chapter 7).

Walking Contemplation

Five to ten minutes per day (add five minutes per week).

Diet

In the first week, choose just one change to make in your diet; for example, switch from 2% milk to fat-free; or, instead of chicken for a main course one day, try a dish made from a soy protein substitute. See Chapter 8 for more suggestions. In week two, make another small change in your diet; if you need to lose weight, determine your calorie count according to your goal weight, and study the sample menus. In week three, make a third small change in your diet and follow one of the sample menus for one or two nonconsecutive days that week. In week four, add a day on your new calorie count and make another small change. Starting in week five, follow the suggested diet for at least five days out of seven.

Some of my students enjoy recording their progress in a chart form. If you like, create a chart or a journal that records your goals for each of the six parts of the program for each week, and include a space to write in how you met your goals, what you experienced during your Fantasy exercises or while meditating, and how you felt about yourself every day. Here is a sample:

Week 1
Exercise

Goal — *warm-ups and 3 exercises.*

Result — *warm-ups only for 2 days, then added the Standing Sun Pose. Felt a little stiff in the back of my legs, but it went away by the end of the week.*

Breathing

Goal — *3 Complete Breath exercises*

Result — *Loved this technique! Found myself doing it while waiting in the doctor's office Wednesday. Helped me feel less nervous.*

Meditation

Goal — *5 minutes*

Result — *Felt like I was just lying there thinking about my "to do" list. About the third day, felt myself stop talking to myself for a few seconds. By the end of the week, I almost fell asleep.*

Fantasy

Goal — *"Vision of Myself"*

Result — *Had trouble seeing anything but a vision of myself crippled up and helpless at first. After a few days, remembered how much better I felt while doing the warm-up exercises and pictured myself straighter and more limber.*

Walking

Goal — *5-10 minutes*

Result — *Got overenthusiastic the first day: walked around the neighborhood for about a half hour - felt sore the next day. Walked 5 minutes anyway. Felt better. Missed only one day this week.*

Diet

Goal — *make one small change in diet*

Result — *Decided to try milk in my tea instead of cream. Succeeded every day except Sunday.*

Always maintain a constant, friendly approach with yourself, reminding yourself that this is a lifetime change that slowly and steadily will build solid supporting blocks of health, strength, and happiness with yourself and your new way of living.

Chapter 3

Yoga Exercise for Arthritis

In this chapter you will find a complete Yoga exercise routine especially designed to be helpful for arthritis. The routine is organized with the easiest exercises presented first, so start at the beginning. If you have not exercised in a long time, I suggest that you begin by practicing only the warm-ups (pages 53-79) and then three additional exercises of your choice. Add one or two exercises each week until you are able to practice the full routine. Try to be regular about practicing every day, but avoid practicing the exercise portion of your routine when your joints are especially swollen, painful, or hot. Exercise when pain and stiffness are at a minimum.

How to Practice Yoga for Best Results

Breathing

It may be tempting to plunge right in and just follow the pictures, but if you do you will miss the important instructions about how to breathe during the exercise. Breathing is a crucial element of Yoga exercises, and each pose or movement has a particular breathing pattern that contributes greatly to its effect. Read once completely through the instructions before beginning, in order to be sure you are breathing correctly as well as to avoid injury.

Always breathe through your nose, both inhaling and exhaling. If you concentrate on the steamlike sound of your breath as you move through the routine, you will notice a wonderful silence in your mind that will naturally lead you into a very restful meditation. (See Chapter 4, p. 112, for how to make the steamlike sound with your breath, and also for suggestions for how to open your breathing passages if they are blocked.)

The exercises have been laid out in a sequence from standing to seated to lying down. The transition between exercises is often where concentration is lost. Try to keep your attention on your breath throughout your entire routine.

Most exercises are movements matched with either an inhalation or an exhalation. You breathe in to a count of three, hold for a count of three, breathe out for a count of three, hold for a count of three, then rest for a count of three. This focuses and settles your mind on the proper position of body, breath, and mind. When holding your breath, you do not have to count slowly; if you find yourself getting winded, increase the speed of your three-count until you feel more comfortable.

Exercise at Your Own Pace

Yoga exercises should not hurt. Be kind to your body; move slowly and carefully, paying attention to how your body feels at all times. I can't stress enough how important it is to exercise at your own pace. As I mentioned previously, if you haven't exercised in a long time, don't try to do the entire routine all at once.

In fact, it's probably a good idea to do only one repetition of each exercise the first few times you try it, just to make sure there is no movement that will aggravate a back condition or other physical problem you may not be aware of. The important thing is to practice at least three exercises every day. When you practice every day, your strength and endurance will gradually increase until you can do the entire routine.

If you find that some of the exercises are too difficult, practice them with only partial movements until you become stronger. Remember, Yoga is a nonviolent practice. If you haven't exercised in a while, you may experience some tightness in your joints and muscles, especially in the back of your legs when you practice forward-bending exercises. With daily practice, you will notice a big difference in your stretching ability in just a few weeks. Many of the exercises are presented with a seated alternative, for those of you who are quite stiff. Start with the seated variation and move into the standing variation when you are stronger. If you are frail, hold on to the back of a sturdy chair when you do the standing exercises.

Most exercises call for about three to five repetitions. Always go at your own pace, remembering that Yoga works best in small steady increments.

Yoga Throughout the Day

If you lead a fairly sedentary lifestyle, you will benefit greatly if you get into the habit of getting up every hour or so and moving around a little. This doesn't mean strenuous or lengthy exercises: just do some simple stretching and bending to increase blood flow to all parts of your body. This habit will also help build strength and flexibility overall, so that your daily Yoga exercise routine becomes easier. Over the course of a day, try to do movements that put all your joints through their full range of motion (the warm-up exercises, pages 53-79, are good range-of-motion movements). Breathe deeply through your nose and imagine the oxygen bringing healing nutrients into the muscles, joints, and bones. Find odd times to fit exercise into your day. For example, many of my students practice warm-up exercises while watching television or talking on the telephone.

The Exercise Sequence

Warm-ups

Warm-up exercises gradually introduce your body to the idea of exercising. In this book, I have increased the usual number of warm-up exercises to provide a full range-of-motion workout for your joints. Warm-ups are simple stretches that work on the major muscle groups of the body, gently stretching the long muscles of the legs and back, gently bending the spine, increasing circulation, and loosening the joints of the shoulders, hips, and spine. Remember to breathe through your nose at all times and concentrate on the sound of the breath. Pay attention to how your body feels, and never do anything that causes pain. In the following routine, the warm-ups begin with the Shoulder Roll and end with the Lazy Stretch (pp. 53-79).

Massage

Following the warm-ups, you will find a detailed section on self-massage. Massage can often relieve joint stiffness. For best results, gently massage a joint before and after exercising it. You can also practice self-massage any time of day to counteract stiffness.

Main Exercise Routine

Instructions for the main Yoga exercise routine begin with the Standing Sun Pose on page 84. The exercises are arranged from standing, to seated, to lying down for easy transition between movements. Remember that many include variations that can be done in a chair if necessary. As I mentioned previously, do not attempt to practice every exercise at once. Begin with all the warm-ups and then follow with two or three exercises of your choice, adding one or more every few days. Your total exercise time should be about 10 to 15 minutes. After several weeks, you can increase this time if you wish. You can substitute new exercises whenever you like without increasing your total daily exercise practice time.

Stress is a pervasive force in our daily lives that can cause us to fear movement. This is especially so when we are afraid of attack, no matter what the source, or whether it's justified or not. It's as if the body feels such a need for protection that it carefully guards its movements so as not to be hurt further. The Shoulder Roll and other warm-ups will help your body to gradually feel more relaxed about the movements that lie ahead in the routine so that it doesn't feel so frightened.

The B-complex vitamins and vitamin C are very important for helping to support your body as it manages stress responses. See Chapter 8 for more information about how to be sure your diet includes enough of these nutrients.

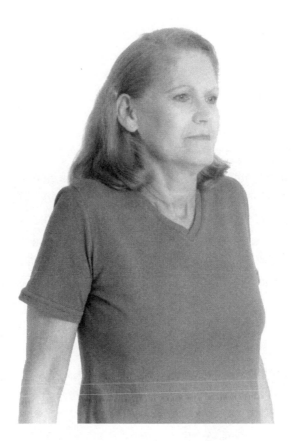

(1) Shoulder Roll

SHOULDER ROLL

Benefits: Loosens shoulder joints and upper back.

Breathe normally throughout this exercise, and always breathe through your nose. Stand with feet parallel and arms hanging loosely at your sides. Lift both shoulders up toward your ears (without bending your elbows) and rotate your shoulders in circles, first forward, then backward, at least 5 times in each direction (1). Keep your arms and hands hanging loosely.

Learning to relax at will is a vital skill for a Yoga student, especially if you have arthritis. Every exercise provides an opportunity to learn a different way to relax your body and mind. Sometimes the best relaxation comes after an exertion. In the Arm Circles, your heart and the rest of your respiratory and circulatory systems are energized, so your entire upper body feels flushed with life-giving blood that is packed with oxygen. Enhance the relaxed feeling by shaking out your arms and shoulders after this exercise.

Sometimes people who have trouble relaxing during the day also have trouble going to sleep at night or staying asleep. If this applies to you, try cutting out caffeinated beverages after 5 pm. Practice a few warm-ups just before bed, and practice two or three Complete Breaths when you lie down. Try to think of nothing except the sound of your breath. Then meditate yourself to sleep with the "I Love You" technique (see page 131).

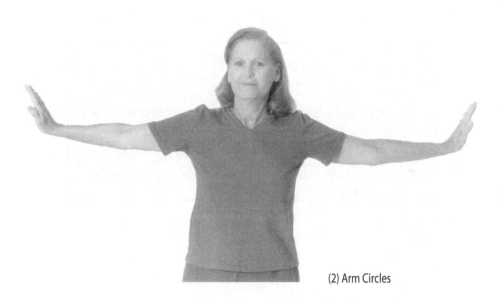

(2) Arm Circles

ARM CIRCLES

Benefits: Increases circulation; strengthens back and shoulders; improves range of motion of shoulders; limbers upper back, chest, and midback.

Stand with feet parallel. Lift your arms straight out to the sides, fingers flexed and palms facing outward (2). Maintaining this position, rotate your arms first in large, slow circles and then in small, faster circles, 5 to 8 times in each direction. Breathe normally throughout. Finish by shaking out arms and shoulders.

In this exercise you are concentrating on the movement of just one part of your body. This is a wonderful opportunity to practice the quiet feeling that you are striving for in meditation. Stop all inner conversation with yourself, which will dilute the effect of the exercise. Instead, imagine as you turn your head slowly that your head is filled with a great silence.

NECK STRETCHES

Benefits: Releases tension in upper back and neck.

Cautions: If you have disk problems in your neck, check with your doctor before trying this exercise.

Breathe normally throughout this exercise. Start by gently bending your neck forward and slightly to the left, so your chin reaches down toward your collarbone. Place your right palm on your neck to monitor the stretch (3). Hold for several seconds, breathing normally. Repeat on the opposite side. Relax your arms and rotate your shoulders a few times to relax your neck muscles, then go on to the following neck stretches:

Slowly turn your head from side to side, as if looking over your shoulder. Next, tilt your head so that your ear drops toward your shoulder (4). Bend three times to each side. Finally, lower your chin toward your chest, then lift your chin until you are looking toward the ceiling (do not drop your head all the way back). Repeat 3 times.

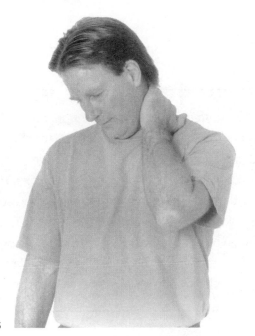

(3) Neck Stretches

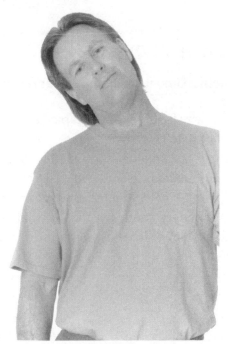

(4) Neck Stretches

The previous warm-ups focused on your upper body. With the Elbow Twist exercise, you will begin to feel the effects of improved circulation in your entire body. Continue the mental exercise described for the Neck Stretches. Imagine yourself filled with a vast silence. Imagine the silence spreading throughout your entire body. You will feel a restful feeling of relief while you slowly twist from side to side. Your physical body will loosen up and begin to lose its fear of movement. Your emotional body will feel centered and focused.

ELBOW TWIST

Benefits: Limbers spine; improves respiration and posture.

Stand with feet a few inches apart, and be sure your back is straight. Raise your arms to chest height, bend your elbows, and place one hand on top of the other. Breathe in completely to a count of three while looking forward, then breathe out slowly to a count of three as you twist toward the left, leading with your left elbow. Look around to the left so your entire upper body is gently twisted (5). Hold for a count of three, then breathe in to a count of three as you return to face front. Repeat 3 times to each side, alternating.

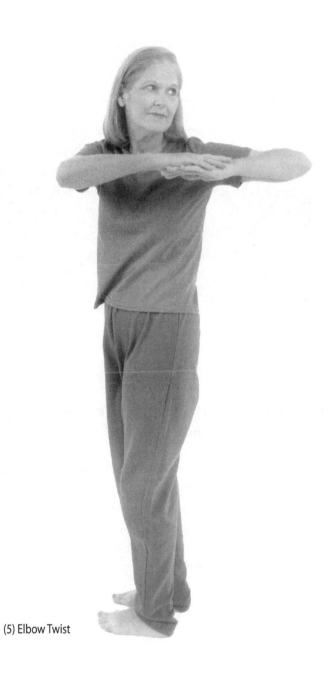

(5) Elbow Twist

You will like this movement. It is an easy exercise to begin with if your body is afraid to move because of pain. It helps give strength to your hands and arms, and you will enjoy the ability to balance on your toes for a moment or two, which is all that is needed. If you are afraid to go up on your toes for fear of falling, hold on to a sturdy chair or kitchen countertop first with one hand, then the other, in order to exercise each side equally.

EASY BALANCE

Benefits: Improves respiration; oxygenates blood; strengthens ankles and calves; improves balance.

Standing with feet parallel and arms at sides, breathe out. Staring at one spot to help maintain balance, breathe in completely to a count of three as you stretch up on your toes and press your fists into your midriff (6). Be sure you are not pressing into your rib cage, but directly below it. Hold for a count of three, then breathe out to a count of three as you relax, lowering your arms and heels. Rest. Repeat 3 times.

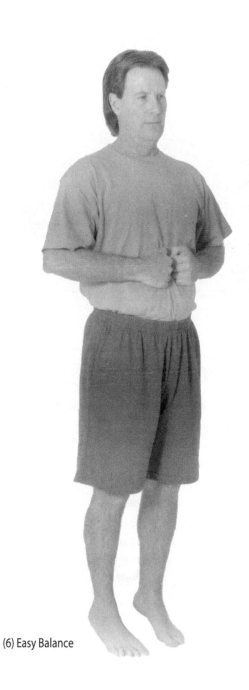

(6) Easy Balance

This is another easy exercise that can be done at any time of day. You can sit on a chair or bed and enjoy the new strength of breathing that this exercise will encourage. It also will help you keep an erect posture by strengthening your back muscles. Try to look steadily at a point in the room without blinking while you do the exercise; this will improve concentration.

ELBOW TOUCH

Benefits: Limbers shoulders and upper back; stretches chest muscles; improves breathing.

Bring the tips of your fingers to the tops of your shoulders and extend your elbows straight out horizontally. Breathe out to a count of three as you slowly bring your elbows forward as if you could touch your elbows together (7). Hold for a count of three. Then breathe in to a count of three as you stretch your elbows back as far as you can comfortably. Hold for a count of three. Repeat for a total of 3 times.

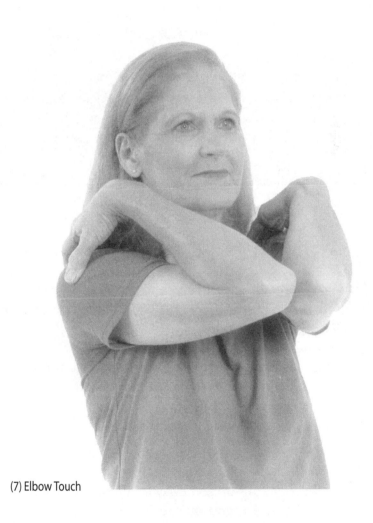

(7) Elbow Touch

The best effect of this exercise is to straighten the spine, freeing the lungs and heart for full intake of fresh oxygen. It will help you gain strength and also contribute to a straight posture and graceful walk. Another important factor in good posture is strong bones and joints. Getting enough calcium in your daily diet will help. See Chapter 8 for more about calcium.

REAR ARM LIFT

Benefits: Improves breathing capacity and heart function by stretching the muscles of the rib cage, chest, and upper back. Improves posture and helps to straighten rounded shoulders.

Cautions: Since lifting your arms to the back is not a common movement, be careful not to strain when doing this exercise for the first time, especially if your shoulders are stiff and sore. It will help to do the Shoulder Massage (see page 81) before and after this exercise.

Stand erect, with hands clasped behind your back. Straighten your arms as much as possible. Breathe out completely. Breathe in to a count of three as you lift your arms up and away from your body, keeping your fingers laced (8). Try not to bend forward, and keep your head erect. Hold your breath in for a count of three, then breathe out and relax to a count of three, lowering your arms to your sides. Rest. Repeat a total of 3 times.

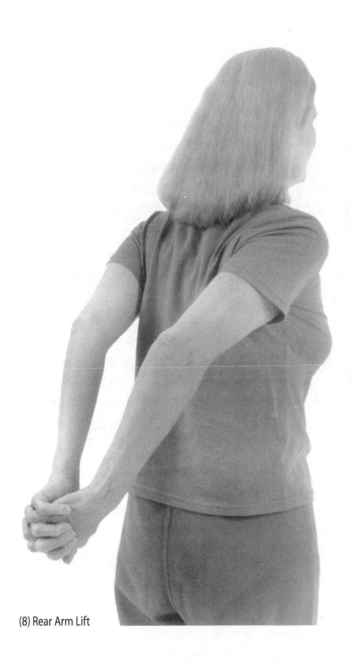

(8) Rear Arm Lift

My teacher Rama used to say that this simple exercise was the key to total body health. It uses all the major muscle groups and affects the nervous, circulatory, glandular, and respiratory systems. Practicing this exercise will prevent the development of a swayback or hunchback. This exercise invites a mystical connection with the sun.

Nothing happens in the physical world without first happening in the mind. If you want to build a chair, for example, you first have to fantasize the chair in your mind; then you pick up the saw and hammer to build the chair. Similarly, when you practice Yoga exercises, you attain best results if you fantasize the changes you want to see in your body. As you practice the Full Bend, use fantasy to visualize your body stretching out until it becomes taut and strong and brave.

FULL BEND AND HOLD
(Paschimottanasan Prep.)

Benefits: Releases tension in upper back and neck; helps to reduce body fat.

Cautions: If you start to feel faint while bending forward, bend only halfway down, but still be sure to let your head, arms, and hands hang forward loosely when you breathe out. Hold on to a chair back or railing with one hand to protect from falling.

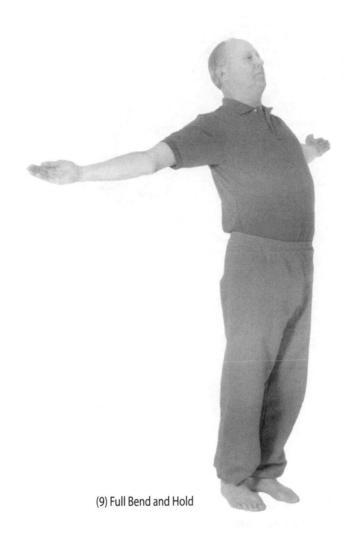

(9) Full Bend and Hold

Stand with feet parallel, a few inches apart. Breathe out completely. Breathe in to a count of three as you slowly raise your arms up and out to your sides, parallel to the floor (9). Stretch back a little as you hold your breath in for a count of three, then breathe out to a count of three as you slowly bend forward, leading with your hands, until you are as far forward as possible. Let your whole body go limp and hold your breath out

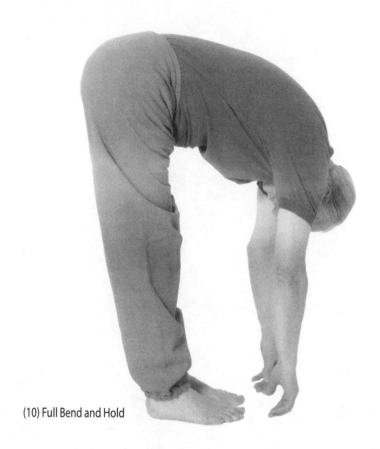

(10) Full Bend and Hold

for a count of three (10). Now breathe in to a count of three as you slowly come back up, bringing your arms out to the sides again. Continue to breathe in as you straighten up, and breathe out as you bend forward, matching your breath to your movement. Repeat 3 to 5 times.

After the last repetition, breathe out and come forward once again, but let your arms relax toward the floor and hold the position, breathing naturally. If you can reach the floor comfortably, let your fingers curl slightly. Just go limp and relax. Let your head hang so your neck stretches. Don't hold your breath. Hold for several seconds, then slowly stand up.

Start your practice of these poses with a chair to assure yourself that you can balance safely. Many times, balance is better on one leg than the other. If this is true in your case, just use a chair to balance when lifting the leg that needs extra help; eventually you will see that your body will balance out with strength on both sides.

Try to feel happy when you do this exercise. Smile and congratulate yourself on your accomplishment as you proudly hold your posture as if in preparation for the dance. This will help fight depression.

Good balance depends on strong bones and a strong nervous system. Getting plenty of the B vitamins will help strengthen your nervous system. See Chapter 8 for suggestions on foods to emphasize for the B-complex vitamins.

LEG LIFTS

Benefits: Limbers hip joints, strengthens legs; improves balance.

Cautions: If your knees or hips are very stiff, painful, or weak, hold on to the back of a sturdy chair with one hand for support while you practice this exercise.

Stand with feet together, hands on your hips. Breathe out. Breathe in to a count of three as you lift your right leg forward, keeping your toes flexed and both legs straight (11). It is more important to keep your legs straight than to lift your leg higher. Hold for a count of three, then breathe out to a count of three and lower the leg. Repeat for a total of 3 times on each leg.

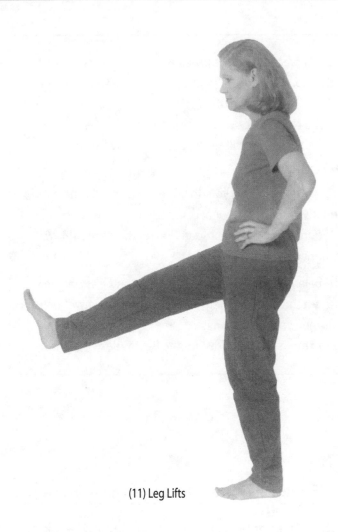

(11) Leg Lifts

Next, breathe in to a count of three as you lift your right leg out to the sides, keeping your toes flexed and your foot pointed forward (12). Hold for a count of three. Breathe out to a count of three and lower the leg. Repeat 3 times on each leg.

Finally, breathe in to a count of three as you lift your right leg back, keeping your toes flexed and both legs straight (13). Hold for a count of three. Breathe out to a count of three and lower. Repeat 3 times on each leg.

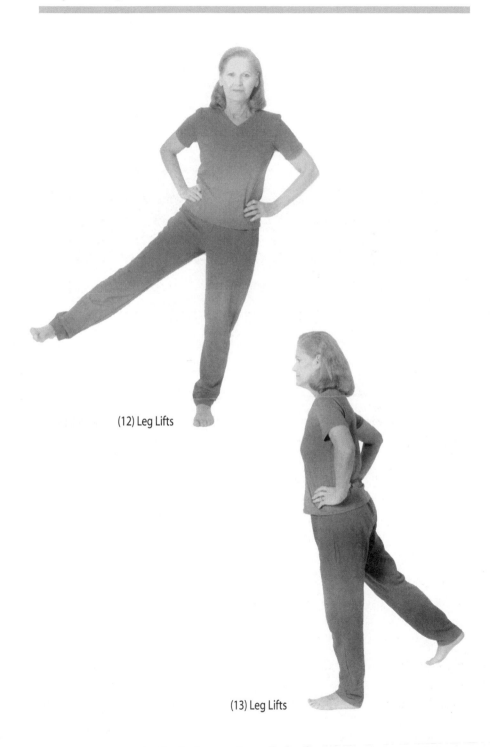

(12) Leg Lifts

(13) Leg Lifts

I have noticed that people with arthritis seldom dance, usually because of the chronic pain and stiffness as well as a fear of movement. Exercises such as the Hip Rotation will help you develop more confidence in movement so that you can try new activities without fear.

HIP ROTATION

Benefits: Limbers lower back and hip joints; increases circulation in pelvic region; gently stretches groin muscles.

Breathe normally throughout this exercise. Stand with feet apart as far as you can comfortably, hands on hips with thumbs forward, so your fingers support your lower back (14). Gently rotate hips forward and back 3 times; then side to side 3 times; then in circles 3 times each direction. Do not strain or pull.

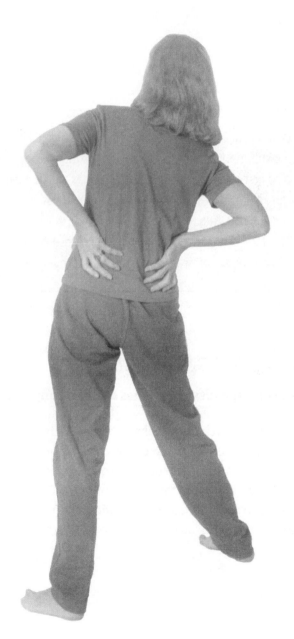

(14) Hip Rotation

Lifting your arms over your head may be difficult if your body has stiffened due to lack of movement. Many people, when they first begin, can lift only a few inches above their hips. I can assure you that if you practice regularly, each week you will notice a little more flexibility, and you will love the feeling of freedom that this achievement brings. Practice in front of a mirror to better appreciate your improvements.

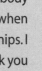

STANDING SIDE STRETCH

Benefits: limbers muscles in the sides and back; improves respiration.

Stand with feet parallel, a few inches apart. Breathe in, then breathe out to a count of three as you reach down toward the floor with your right arm and simultaneously reach up toward the ceiling and over your head with your left arm (15). Hold for a count of three. Breathe in to a count of three as you return to your starting position, then breathe out to a count of three as you bend toward the left. Repeat 3 times on each side, alternating.

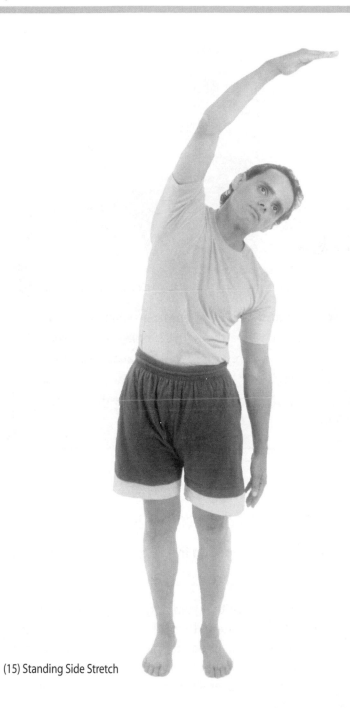

(15) Standing Side Stretch

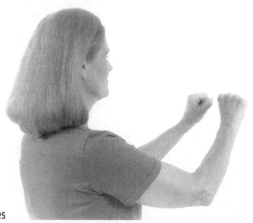

(16) Hand Limbering Exercises

Staying independent is important for everyone, and especially for people with arthritis. This simple exercise, which you can do all day long, will keep your hands flexible and strong so that you can open jars, play the piano, have fun in the garden, or do whatever activity you like without pain or stiffness.

HAND LIMBERING EXERCISES

Benefits: improves range of motion in wrists and finger joints, making everyday tasks easier.

You can practice this exercise either standing or sitting comfortably. Make fists of your hands (16), then extend them (17). Repeat several times. Press your fingers together as if making a steeple (18). Press back on the fingers of one hand, using your other hand (19). Repeat on the other side. Rotate your wrists in circles, several times each direction. Now shake out your arms and hands, and relax.

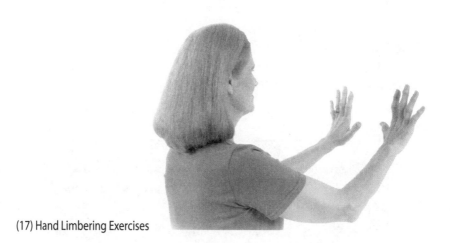

(17) Hand Limbering Exercises

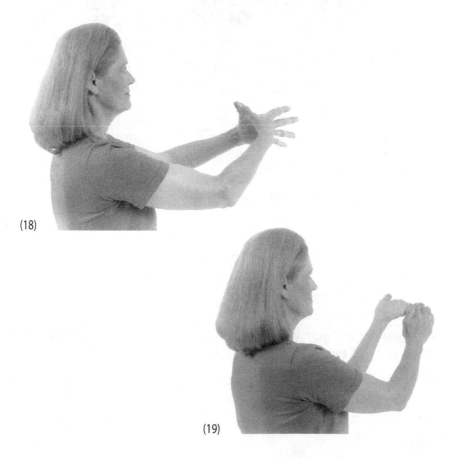

(18)

(19)

When my great teacher Lakshmanjoo was teaching me about the Yogic ethic of Tolerance, he said that a true hero is the person who can take one more step. Practicing Yoga techniques every day will build your endurance and courage so you can keep going no matter what happens. The Lazy Stretch exercise is particularly beneficial for improving lung capacity, balance, and stamina, giving your physical body the support it needs to remain strong.

LAZY STRETCH

Benefits: Stretches back of legs and lower back; strengthens ankles and calves; improves respiration.

Stand with feet shoulder width apart. Bend your knees and rest your forearms on your knees with hands clasped. Breathe in to a count of three and look up, arching your back slightly (20). Hold for a count of three. Breathe out to a count of three as you straighten your legs while keeping your forearms on your knees (21). Tuck your chin toward your chest. Repeat 3 to 5 times.

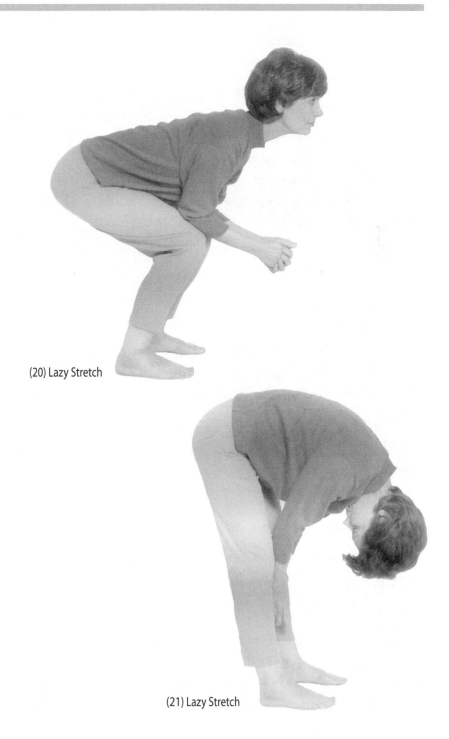

(20) Lazy Stretch

(21) Lazy Stretch

> Self-massage has lasting benefits. It is particularly helpful in improving circulation, which helps prevent damage to the joints, especially those of the fingers, knees, and ankles. You can practice massage anytime you are sitting comfortably, such as while watching television. Keep a bottle of lotion near your chair to increase the pleasant experience.

MASSAGE

Benefits: Helps remove stiffness in the joints and muscles and improves circulation, making exercise easier and more pleasant, and reducing strain and injury. Helps keep you in touch with your physical body, which leads to greater self-esteem.

The point of these exercises is not to press hard with the hands and fingers but simply to increase warmth in the affected area. Use your whole hand – primarily the palm – when rubbing a joint, not just your fingers. Each joint should be massaged for at least 15 seconds. These exercises can be done throughout the day as needed.

Shoulders: Start by supporting your right elbow in your left hand. With your right hand, gently rub your left shoulder (22) using your whole hands, not just the fingers. Rub the entire joint for 15 to 30 seconds. Repeat on the right side.

Elbow: Massage your elbows, one at a time, with the opposite hand (23). Rub the entire elbow joint for 15 to 30 seconds.

Neck: Rub the right side and back of your neck with your right hand (24). Use your palm, and rub for 15 to 30 seconds. Repeat on the left side.

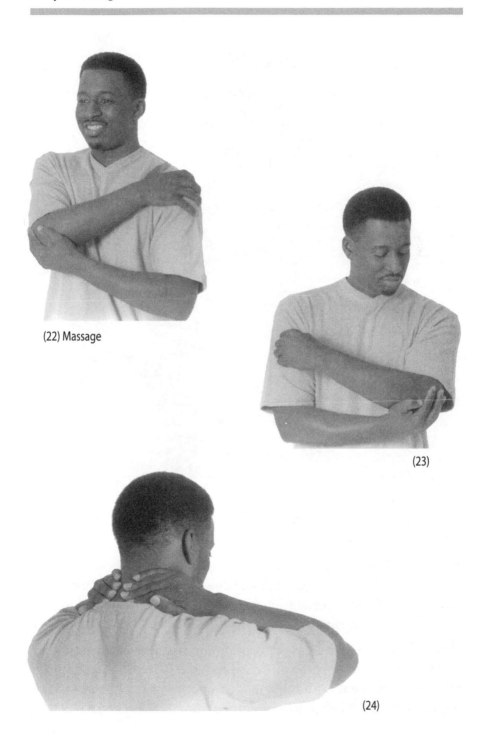

(22) Massage

(23)

(24)

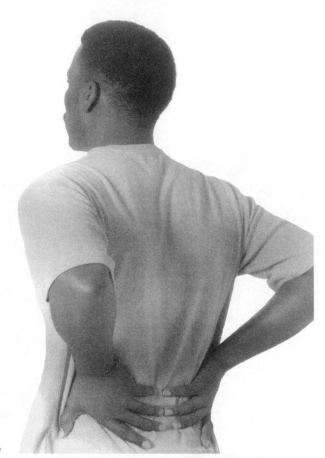

(25) Massage

Lower back: Place both hands on your lower back and rub firmly up and down all the way to the tailbone, using your palms (25).

Knees and ankles: Massage one knee at a time. Place both hands on your knee. Rub up with one hand and down with the other hand simultaneously in a semicircular motion over the entire knee area (26). Use your palm. Massage ankles similarly.

Fingers: Starting at the base of your thumb, use your opposite thumb and fingers to rub firmly in a circular motion all over and around the joint. Move up the thumb, rubbing the same way at each knuckle joint. Repeat with each of your fingers, starting from the base of each (27).

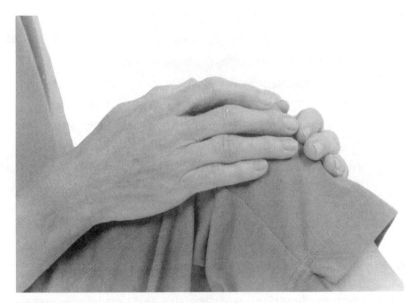

(26) Massage

(27) Massage

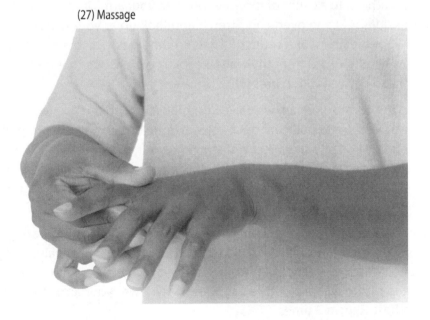

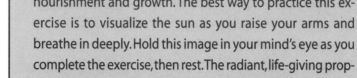

This exercise is called the Sun Pose because it brings radiant, all-around health, just as the sun is the earth's source for nourishment and growth. The best way to practice this exercise is to visualize the sun as you raise your arms and breathe in deeply. Hold this image in your mind's eye as you complete the exercise, then rest. The radiant, life-giving properties of the sun will fill your heart and body.

STANDING SUN POSE (Padahasthasan)

Benefits: Improves functioning of digestive and circulatory systems; exercises heart and lungs; limbers and strengthens legs and back.

Stand with feet parallel. Keep your knees straight but not locked. Breathe out. Breathe in to a count of three as you raise your arms in a wide circle to the sides (28) and overhead. Stretch and look up at your hands (29). Hold your breath in for a count of three. Breathe out to a count of three as you bend forward from the waist, keeping your hands together and your head between your arms (30).

Grasp the back of your ankles, calves, or thighs firmly, bend your elbows, tuck your chin, and pull your torso toward your legs (31). Be sure to pull by bending your elbows instead of straining your lower back. Keep your knees straight and hold your breath out for a count of three. [NOTE: If you have back or neck problems, bend only halfway down, and do not pull your torso in.]

Release and breathe in to a count of three as you slowly straighten, bringing your arms in a wide circle to the sides and over your head again. Look up and stretch as in photo 29. Hold your breath in for a count of three. Breathe out to a count of three as you slowly lower your arms to your sides. Rest. Repeat 3 times.

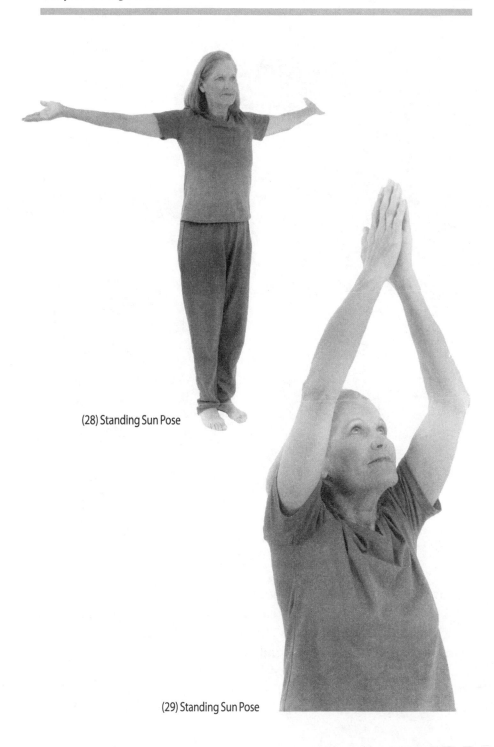

(28) Standing Sun Pose

(29) Standing Sun Pose

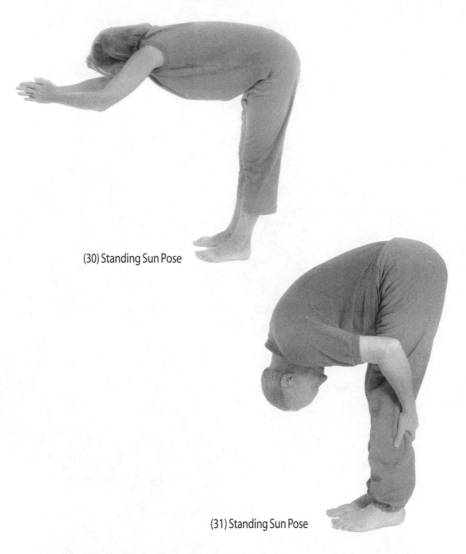

(30) Standing Sun Pose

(31) Standing Sun Pose

Variation: If you are not able to reach over your head, or if your balance is shaky, you may do this exercise seated in a sturdy chair. Sit with your hips pressing against the back of the chair and separate your knees, with feet flat. Make sure your feet are firmly braced. Follow the breathing and movement instructions as above, lifting as high as you can with your arms, and reaching down toward the floor between your legs toward the floor instead of grasping your legs as in the standing version.

In Yoga, the nervous system is often pictured figuratively as covered with an inhibiting, mucuslike covering that contributes to feelings of sluggishness, dullness, and imbalance. Exercises such as the Whirlwind create an internal heat that clears away this obstruction so the nervous system becomes bright and active. You will feel this heat in your body as you practice; you'll also probably notice a more positive and energetic state of mind.

THE WHIRLWIND (Nauli)

Benefits: Compresses internal abdominal organs; strengthens abdominal muscles; reduces body fat. Many people feel a very pleasant warmth building up during the exercise.

Caution: Do not practice the standing variation if you have a lower back problem, as it puts greater strain on your back when standing.

Because this exercise requires you to hold your breath out for quite a while, it can be a bit strenuous until you learn it. Be sure to read through the entire set of instructions before beginning. An excellent warm-up exercise, which will strengthen your abdominal muscles, is an Easy Sit-up: Lie on your back with arms at your sides and knees bent. Breathe in, then breathe out as you stretch your hands toward your knees, using your stomach muscles to lift your head and shoulders. Breathe in and relax back to the starting position. Practice this for a few weeks until your strength increases. If you can easily do 15 to 20 sit-ups in a row, you should be able to perform the Rising Breath and Whirlwind exercises without straining.

Begin with a technique called the Rising Breath *(Uddhyana)*. It is very beneficial to health, strength, and brightness of mind, and it will help you master the movement needed for the Whirlwind.

Sitting on the very edge of a sturdy chair, separate your knees and "plant" your feet flat on the floor. Place your hands just above your knees, pointing in. Tuck your chin into your throat. Begin by taking five deep and strong Belly Breaths (see p. 114), then breathe out forcefully and completely. Be sure all the air is expelled. Holding your breath out, suck in your abdominal muscles back toward your spine and up toward your diaphragm (32). Hold for just a moment, then release your stomach muscles, release your breath, breathe in, and relax. Relax and rest until your breath returns to normal. Practice 3 repetitions.

When you feel relatively proficient in this movement, go on to the Whirlwind *(Nauli)*, which is a similar contraction that you learn to move from side to side in your abdominal cavity. Begin in the same seated position, with chin tucked into your chest. Breathe in deeply, then breathe out forcefully and completely. Hold your breath out and suck in your abdominal muscles back toward your spine and up toward your diaphragm. Press down slightly on your left leg and you will feel the left side of your abdominal wall contract. Now press equally with both hands and then with the right hand only. You will feel the abdominal contraction move across the front of your belly from left to right. Now equalize the pressure on your knees and slowly let your belly relax. Relax your breath and your entire body.

For daily practice, start with one repetition and work up to five. Each repetition consists of left to center to right and back to center. Don't hold any of the positions for more than a few seconds. Always relax completely between repetitions. As you get stronger, you can do up to three cycles during each repetition. Be gentle with yourself. Rest immediately if you feel dizziness or discomfort.

Variation: For a more challenging variation of this exercise, practice in a standing, half-squat position, with hands on separated knees as instructed above. In this position, the pose has very powerful effects on the reproductive system as the abdominal muscles are pulled in and up.

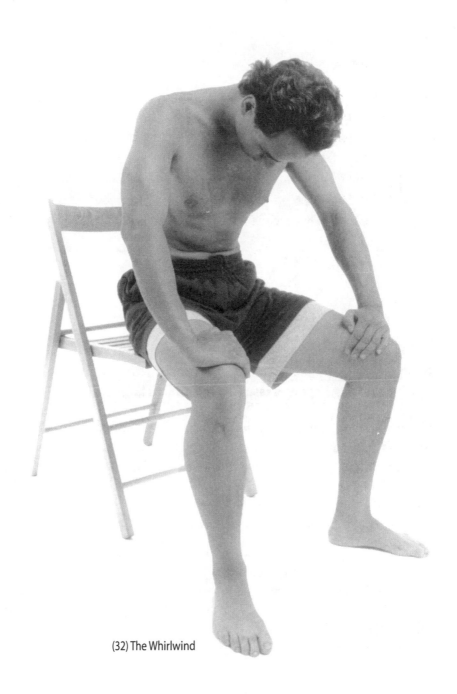

(32) The Whirlwind

This exercise looks like a rest pose, but it is actually a very powerful technique for bringing all the parts of yourself into harmony. Gather yourself together internally as you strongly compress your body as much as you can without discomfort. Stop inner conversation. Try to stay silent in your mind. My teacher told me this poses increases intuition.

BABY POSE (Virasan Var.)

Benefits: Limbers and relaxes lower back; improves circulation to the brain and pelvic region; improves functioning of reproductive and digestive systems; improves respiration; reduces large stomach.

Sit on your feet with knees together. Slowly bend forward so your head touches the floor (33). This will relax your shoulders and neck. Your head can rest on the forehead, bridge of the nose, or top of head. Settle yourself into the most comfortable position you can find. Let your breath relax, and hold for as long as you can comfortably. If this position is impossible, try resting your head on folded arms (34).

Variation: If your hips or knees are too stiff to practice this position on the floor, you may practice it seated in a sturdy chair with hips pressed against the back of the chair. Bend forward from the waist over your knees. Let your arms and head hang loosely so that you receive the same benefits of compression and relaxation (35).

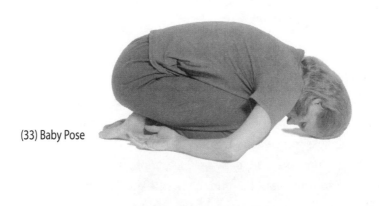

(33) Baby Pose

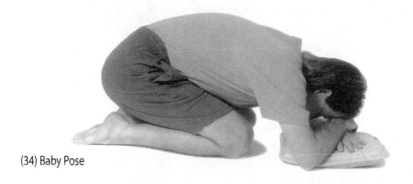

(34) Baby Pose

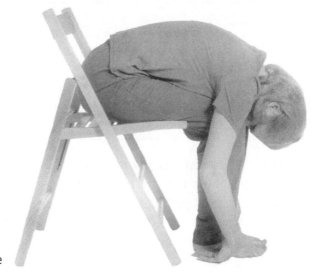

(35) Baby Pose

You've probably noticed that some Yoga exercises (asans) are named for animals. Some people think this is because the pose looks somewhat like that animal. This is only partly correct. In Yoga, asans are done not just for physical effects but also to understand and identify with the beautiful, healthful qualities of the animals, mythological beings, or phenomena they are named for. These qualities rest in the collective unconscious, which has been with us from ancient times. Earlier I suggested that you think of yourself absorbing the energizing, life-giving qualities of the sun while doing the Sun Pose. When you practice the Cat Breath, you take on the graceful, flexible qualities of a cat. The arching movement of this exercise presses on the thyroid gland in the neck, helping to ensure normal weight as well as balanced body systems.

CAT BREATH

Benefits: Limbers lower and midback; tightens stomach muscles; improves breathing.

Start on hands and knees. Breathe in to a count of three as you arch your back and look up (36), feeling the stretch in your chest and neck. Hold for a count of three, then breathe out to a count of three as you round your back and pull up on your stomach, stretching the entire length of your spine (37). Tuck your chin and hold for a count of three. Relax and rest. Repeat 3 times.

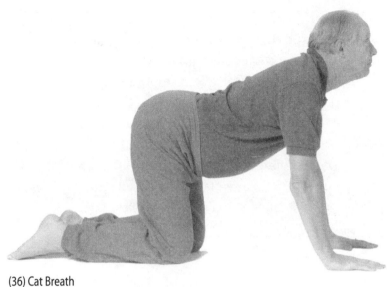

(36) Cat Breath

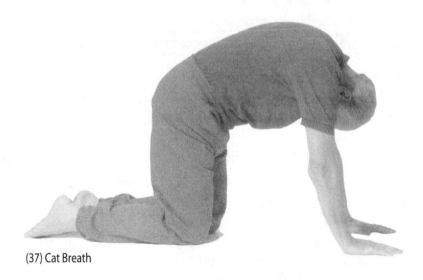

(37) Cat Breath

Variation: If you cannot rest on your knees, you can do this exercise seated on the edge of a chair with hands braced on knees.

When you practice Yoga regularly, you become flexible not only physically, but also emotionally. Being emotionally flexible means that you learn to be more tolerant of change and less judgmental of yourself and others. Once I asked my teacher Lakshmanjoo why Yogis love water so much, and he told me that it is because water has no resistance. People who develop flexibility of mind and body are not troubled by the pain of resistance; they move with a silken grace and take on a youthful and beautiful appearance.

SPINE TWIST (Ardha Matsyendrasan)

Benefits: Improves digestion; limbers and tones entire spine; strengthens and limbers rib cage; relieves chronic constipation; helps relieve bladder, urinary tract, and prostate problems; improves circulation.

Sit up with both legs bent in front of you. Bend your left knee and lay it on the floor with your left foot under your right knee. Pick up your right foot and carry it across your left knee (38). Pull your left foot in close to your body.

Turn toward the right and bring your left arm over your right knee. With your left elbow, press your right knee back as far as it will go (39), then straighten your left arm and grasp the right big toe. If you can't reach your toe, grasp your ankle or knee instead. Bring your right hand close in to your body, fingers pointed in, and straighten the arm. Straighten your back, breathe in to a count of three looking forward, then breathe out to a count of three as you twist toward the right as far as you can (40). Look at a spot on the wall just above eye level. Hold your breath out for a count of three. Release, relax, and repeat on the opposite side. This exercise is done only once on each side.

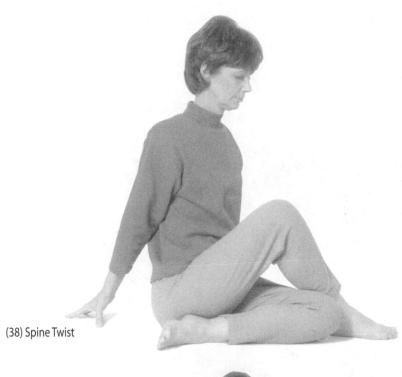

(38) Spine Twist

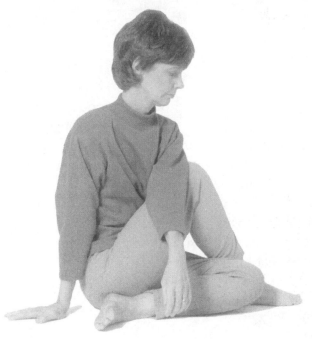

(39) Spine Twist

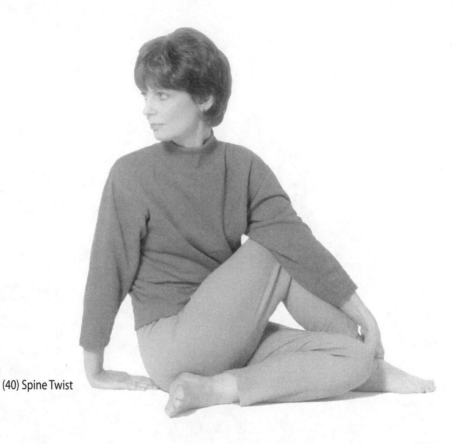

(40) Spine Twist

Variation: For a less-strenuous pose, keep the left leg outstretched (41), or practice the exercise in a chair (42): Seated in a sturdy chair without leaning back, straighten your back and place your right hand on the outside of your left knee. Reach around the back of the chair with your left arm and hold firmly. Breathe in to a count of three with back straight, then breathe out to a count of three as you turn to face left, using your arms as leverage to twist a little further. Hold your breath out for a count of three, then breathe in to a count of three as you return to your starting position. Repeat 3 times.

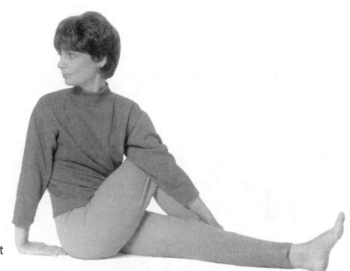

(41) Spine Twist

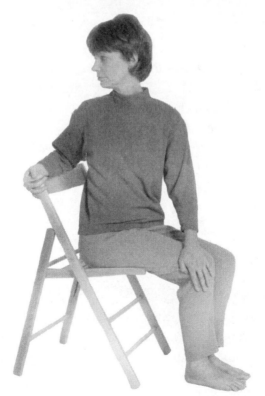

(42) Spine Twist

Don't underestimate the importance of simple movements such as the Foot Flap and Ankle Rotation. These exercises will help strengthen your legs and make them beautiful, too. In Yoga, it doesn't matter how easy or difficult an exercise is; what matters is your attention to the details and your commitment to daily practice.

You might enjoy a story that Rama told me in India. Once when he was walking near the burning ghats (cremation grounds) in Ludhiana, in the Punjab near the northern border of India, he saw a line of people carrying a litter with a body on it toward the fires. Rama said that for some reason he went up to the group and asked who this person was and why the death had occurred. They told him it was a young woman who had died after a long illness.

Rama stepped closer and pulled the shroud away from her face. He saw right away that she was not dead, but in a coma, and he turned the whole procession around and took the girl on the litter back to his residence. Somehow (it was never clear to me how), Rama was able to revive her. She opened her eyes and he bent over her and said, "Do you want to live?" She was able to say yes, and then he sent all the procession home and kept the girl there in his compound. He then told me how he asked her to breathe in and make a fist; that was her beginning of the exercise that brought her back to health. The young lady lived and prospered, even spending time in the jungle camp with Rama and me at Saptasarovar, above Haridwar on the Ganges.

My point in telling you this story is to encourage you to try even the smallest movement with the breath to encourage your return to health. It is not necessary to be able to do all the exercises at first try.

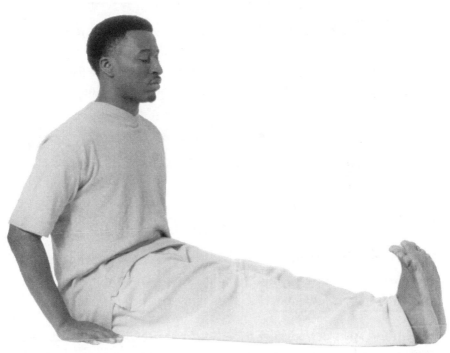

(43) Foot Flap and Ankle Rotation

FOOT FLAP AND ANKLE ROTATION

Benefits: Limbers and strengthens ankle and calf muscles, and improves circulation in the extremities.

Sit up straight with legs outstretched. Push your toes forward and pull them back (43), several times, stretching as far as possible in each direction. Now rotate each ankle in turn, three times in one direction, then three times in the other direction, This exercise can be done sitting on the edge of a chair, with heels resting on the floor, legs straight; sitting in bed supported by the headboard; or lying in bed.

The two bodies, physical and emotional/spiritual, are symbolized in Yoga philosophy by two triangles, one pointing upward and the other pointing downward. When the two are superimposed one on the other, they make a star shape. In the Diamond Pose, your body makes that shape. Visualize this star as you practice the Diamond Pose.

DIAMOND POSE (Shiva Shaktiasan)

Benefits: Tones and strengthens entire nervous system; strengthens and stretches the sciatic nerve; improves digestion; strengthens and limbers hip joints; limbers lower back.

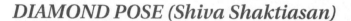

Sit with the soles of your feet together, knees relaxed outward, hands clasped around your toes. Breathe in to a count of three as you straighten your back (44), then breathe out to a count of three as you bend forward, bringing your head toward your feet and letting your elbows fall outside your knees (45). Tuck your chin into your throat, contract your rectal muscles, and hold your breath out for a count of three. Breathe in and release. Rest. Repeat 3 times.

To limber hips and knees, grasp ankles instead of feet. Breathe in to a count of three, then breathe out to a count of three and bend forward, keeping your back straight and pressing your elbows on your thighs to increase the stretch (46). Hold for a count of three. Release, rest, and repeat.

Variation: If you cannot bend one knee, keep that leg outstretched and bend the opposite knee, so that the foot rests inside your opposite knee or thigh. Grasp the toes of that foot with both hands and breathe and bend as instructed above.

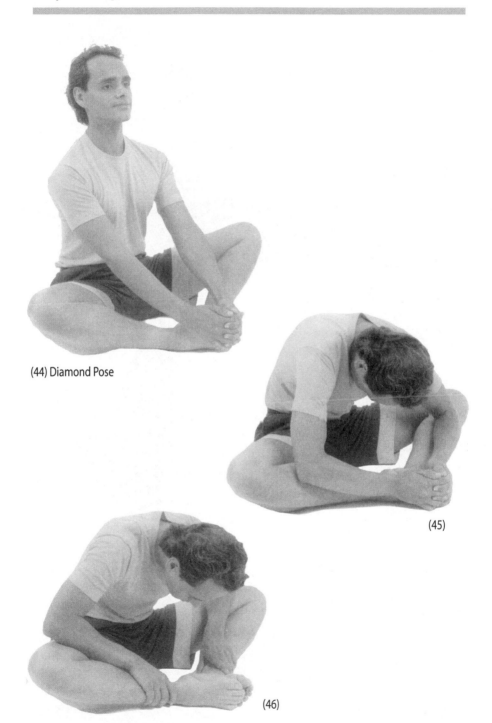

(44) Diamond Pose

(45)

(46)

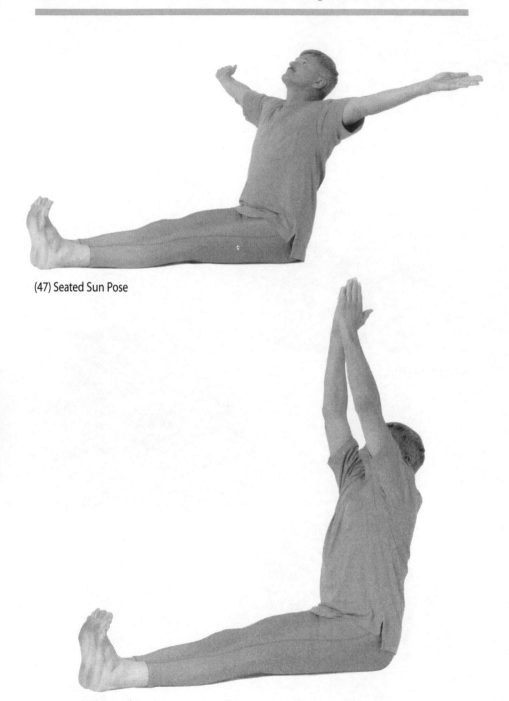

(47) Seated Sun Pose

(48) Seated Sun Pose

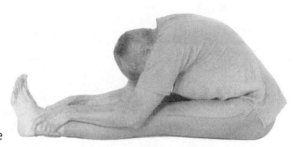

(49) Seated Sun Pose

This Sun Pose is very effective in providing energy and health to the body. Visualize the sun as you practice it, just as you do with the Standing Sun Pose. As you become more proficient in this exercise, you will become aware of more graceful movements, and your posture will improve greatly. When you are struggling with joint pain, good posture can help you look and feel better instantly. This exercise has long-lasting effects on the straightness and lengthening of the spine. I practiced this exercise every day in the early years of my Yoga practice, and I grew three inches after the age of 35!

SEATED SUN POSE (Paschimottanasan)

Benefits: Stretches back of legs; limbers and strengthens lower back; massages internal organs.

Bring both legs straight out in front of you and flex your toes. Sit straight, breathe out to a count of three with arms at your sides, then breathe in to a count of three as you raise your arms in a wide circle to the sides (47) and overhead. Press your palms together, look up, and stretch from the rib cage (48). Visualize the sun. Hold your breath in for a count of three.

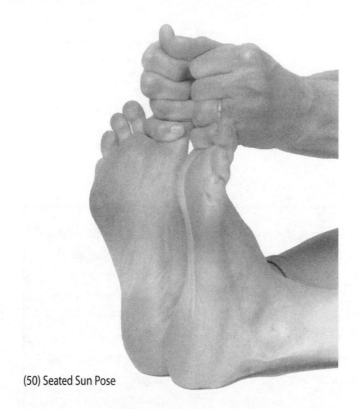

(50) Seated Sun Pose

Breathe out to a count of three as you bend forward, tucking your chin toward your chest. Grasp your ankles, bend your elbows, and pull your torso toward your legs (49). Remember to pull by bending your arms, not by pushing with your lower back. Hold your breath out for a count of three.

If you are limber enough to reach your feet (and still bend your elbows), grasp your big toes as shown (50).

Release and breathe in to a count of three, bringing your arms to the sides and over your head again. Stretch and look up as before. Breathe out to a count of three as you bring your arms back down to your sides. Rest and relax. Repeat 3 times.

Variation: This exercise may also be done sitting up in bed with legs outstretched, back supported by the headboard.

Many exercises, such as this one, help to stimulate your thyroid gland by stretching your neck, which brings a wonderful balance to your body's systems. This exercise also illustrates the important Yogic principle of rest and exertion. When you practice any Yoga exercise, make the exertion with your full attention, and then rest with your full attention. Resting with full attention means completely relaxing all your muscles, bones, and joints, your breathing, and your thoughts as well. Focus on the feeling of stillness, inside and out.

EASY COBRA (Bhujangasan Var.)

Benefits: Gently limbers entire spine; balances both halves of body; improves circulation, massages all internal organs, helps increase lung capacity.

Cautions: Do not do this exercise if you have had recent surgery, especially abdominal surgery.

Lie on your stomach resting on your forearms with hands clasped and elbows on the floor just below your shoulders, fairly close to your body. Breathe out and let your head and upper back relax forward (51). Now breathe in to a count of three as you lift your head and eyes up and back

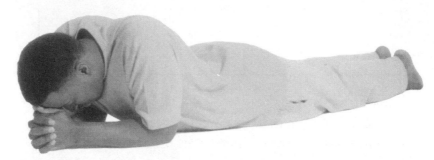

(51) Easy Cobra

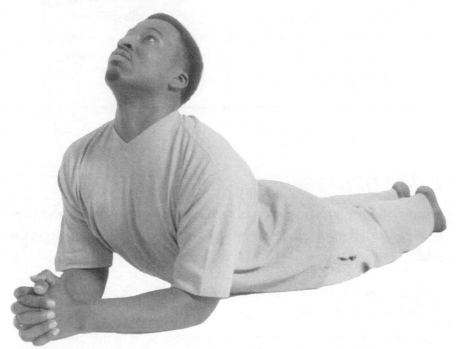

(52) Easy Cobra

as far as possible without strain, then arching your back and stretching up on your elbows, so you feel a slight stretch along your entire spinal column (52). Do not strain. Hold for a count of three and do not blink as you look up through your forehead. Breathe out to a count of three as you relax your back, then your head and eyes, until your forehead returns to your clasped hands. Rest. Repeat 3 times.

Yoga exercise places a great emphasis on strengthening the back muscles and spinal column, because your back is the support of your entire body. At least 20% of adults develop some kind of chronic back pain. Usually the cause can be traced to years of inactivity as well as unsafe lifting and carrying habits. The Boat Pose will strengthen your back muscles very effectively. The compression on the stomach acts as a stimulus to digestion. This exercise also helps to reduce appetite.

You are probably aware that eating a greater amount of fiber can help improve digestion. But did you know that fiber also acts as an appetite suppressant? Because your body has to use more energy to break down the fiber, it takes a greater number of calories to process fiber-rich foods than foods that are low in fiber.

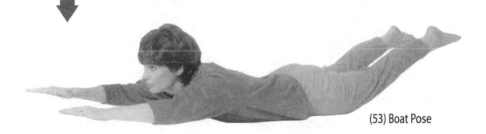

(53) Boat Pose

BOAT POSE (Poorva Navasan)

Benefits: Strengthens back muscles; improves digestion and functioning of all internal organs.

Lie on your stomach, forehead to the floor and arms stretched out in front. Breathe out to a count of three, then breath in to a count of three and lift your arms, legs, and head (53). Look up. Hold your breath for a count of three, then breathe out to a count of three as you lower to your starting position. Rest. Repeat 3 times.

Variation: If you are experiencing stiffness or pain in your back, begin by lifting only one arm at a time, using the complete breath instructions, then one leg, then both legs, both arms, and finally arms, legs, and head together.

I used to pretend that this compression exercise was actually pumping illness and pain out of my body. I wanted to feel that I was able to help myself get well, and doing this made me feel better. I highly recommend that you observe your mental attitude while you practice all these exercises. Refuse hopeless, sad thoughts while you practice. If you notice this type of thought slipping into your mind, replace it at once with positive, helpful conversation that will help lead you out of depression. Day by day you will benefit from this and help yourself to be the person you want to be.

KNEE SQUEEZE

Benefits: Improves digestion; limbers and relaxes lower back and hips; improves circulation in pelvic region; removes metabolic waste products from the body.

Lie on your back with arms overhead and legs together. Breathe out completely to a count of three. Breathe in to a count of three as you bend your left knee and grasp it with both hands, bringing it in toward your chest, then squeeze your knee to your chest and lift your forehead up toward your knee (54). Hold your breath in for a count of three. Relax and breathe out to a count of three as you lower your head, arms, and legs down to the floor back to your starting position. Repeat with the left leg, then twice more on each side, alternating. Rest if needed between repetitions.

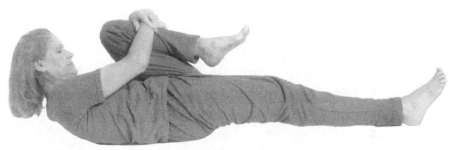

(54) Knee Squeeze

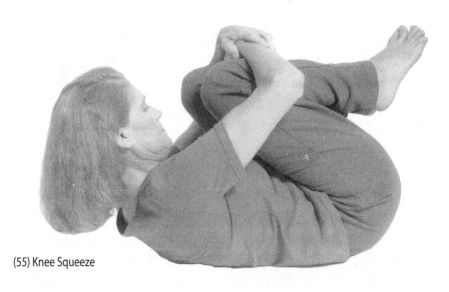

(55) Knee Squeeze

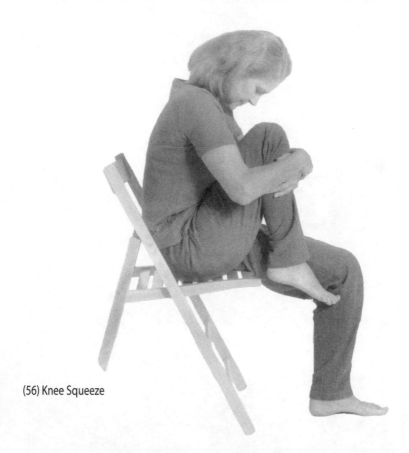

(56) Knee Squeeze

Rest a moment, then do the same movement with both legs at the same time. Hold your breath in for a count of three as you try to touch your forehead to your knees (55). Breathe out to a count of three and relax back to your starting position. Rest. Repeat 3 times.

Variation 1: If you have arthritis in your knees, grasp under the knee, around your upper thigh, instead of the knee itself.

Variation 2: If you have difficulty getting on the floor, this exercise may be done in bed. You can also practice a variation of this exercise sitting in a sturdy chair. Sit on the edge of the chair with your back straight, breathe out, then breathe in, lift one knee, wrap your arms around the knee and squeeze, holding your breath in and dropping your forehead toward your knee (56). Then breathe out and release. Repeat 3 times with each leg, alternating.

Chapter 4

Yoga Breathing Techniques for Arthritis

Your Seated Position

Establishing a comfortable, erect seated position is essential for learning this technique. You have several options; be assured that you don't have to get into a complicated cross-legged position in order to benefit from breathing techniques. If you are quite stiff, or when you are first learning the technique, just sit on the edge of a straight chair, with your feet flat on the floor or toes tucked under slightly (57). Do not lean against the back of the chair. Rest your hands on your knees.

If your hips and knees are fairly limber, you can try sitting on the floor, either kneeling or sitting cross-legged (58). If you sit cross-legged, be sure to use one or more firm cushions to raise your hips as shown in the photo. This will keep your lower back and stomach from becoming tense, which usually results in

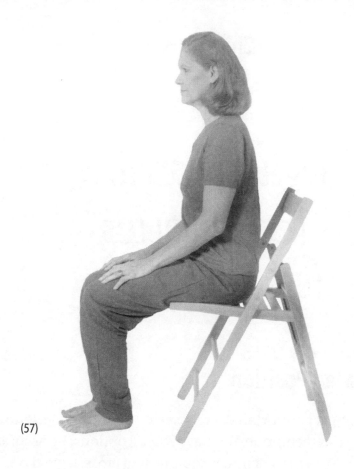

(57)

slouching. In order for the breathing techniques to work, your back must remain straight and relaxed.

Always Breathe Through Your Nose

Always inhale and exhale through your nose — never your mouth. This is important in regulating the speed of your breath and improving your concentration. It helps to focus on the sound of your breath. If you close your throat slightly, you will hear a

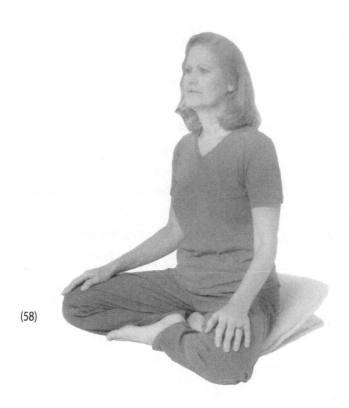

(58)

steamlike sound as you breathe in and out. Concentrating on this sound will help you keep your attention on your breath.

If one side of your nose is blocked, try this technique for opening it: If the right side is blocked, place your right fist in your left armpit and hold for a few minutes until the right side opens. Reverse the procedure to open the opposite side. Another method is to simply lie on your side for a few minutes: if the right nostril is blocked, lie on your left side. If neither of these techniques works, just do the best you can. Remember that although breathing through both nostrils equally is the ideal, you can still practice if your nose is partially blocked. The longer you practice Yoga, the more these passages will open.

When to Practice Breathing

When you are first starting to practice, do a few Complete Breath exercises at the beginning of your routine to help you get in the mood to practice and help you detach your mind from any cares or anxieties that you may be experiencing. Make the other breathing techniques in this section a part of your routine, preferably just before you lie down for meditation. You can also use breathing exercises — particularly the Complete Breath — any time of day to help calm stressful feelings you may be experiencing, to help manage pain, or to change your thinking pattern. You can practice almost anywhere: lying in bed, in the car while waiting for a light to change (please do not practice while actively driving), in a waiting room at the bank or doctor's office, or standing in line.

Belly Breath

Place your hands loosely on your belly below your navel. Breathe in through your nose and relax your belly as you imagine that you are filling your belly with air, expanding it and pushing your hands outward. This movement will relax all your internal organs and cause the diaphragm to drop to its fullest extent, allowing the air to reach the bottom section of your lungs. Breathe out now, through your nose, and slowly, consciously, contract your belly muscles, pushing in with your hands until all the air is out. Repeat several times. Do not hold your breath at any time. Remember: as you inhale the belly expands outward; as you exhale the belly contracts inward.

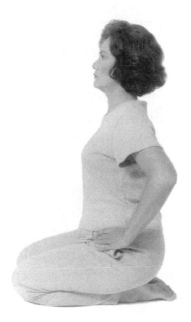

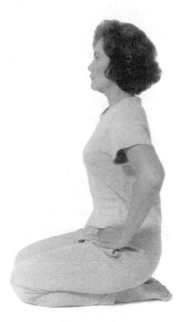

(59) Complete Breath   (60) Complete Breath

Complete Breath

In the Complete Breath, the movement of the Belly Breath is extended up into your ribs, where you expand the muscles between your ribs, and finally your chest, where you push air into the topmost sections of your lungs. Always breathe through your nose, and concentrate on the sound of the breath as described earlier.

Place your hands on your belly or hips and breathe out, trying not to slouch forward. Tighten your belly muscles to get as much air out as possible. Now begin to breathe in from the bottom up, letting your belly muscles relax so the air appears to fill your belly.

Continue to breathe in and feel the air filling the center part of your torso. Imagine the muscles between your ribs stretching so that your ribs expand in all directions, not just forward.

Breathe in a little more and feel the air filling the very top sections of your lungs (59). Do not hold your breath, but gently start to breathe out, slowly, from the top down. First relax your chest, then let your ribs contract, and finally tighten your belly and push the last of the air out (60). Do not hold your breath at the bottom of the cycle either. Repeat the Complete Breath three to ten times.

Depending on your current breath capacity, the complete cycle of the Complete Breath (one inhalation, one exhalation) may take 10 to 30 seconds. It is important to breathe in and out for approximately the same length of time. Most of us naturally breathe out longer than we breathe in. In the Complete Breath you are counteracting that tendency and breathing more evenly.

Alternate Nostril Breath

The main purpose for this breathing technique is to balance the two halves of the body and the two bodies, the physical and spiritual.

In a comfortable seated position or in a chair, curl the first and second fingers of your right hand inward, holding them down with the fleshy part of your thumb. The third and fourth fingers should remain extended. Close your right nostril with your thumb (61), and breathe in through the left nostril only. Hold for a count of three, then close the left nostril with your third and fourth fingers (62), open the right, and breathe out, hold for a count of three, then in again, through the right nostril. Continue alternating by breathing out, then in, through one side at a time, holding for a count of three at each transition from inhalation to exhalation. Repeat 5 to 10 times.

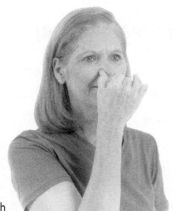

(61) Alternate Nostril Breath

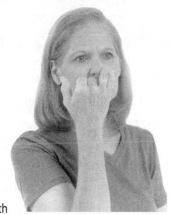

(62) Alternate Nostril Breath

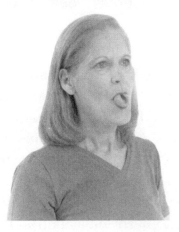

(63) Cooling Breath

The Cooling Breath *(Sitali)*

This technique has a cooling effect on the body; it also improves resistance to disease and enhances physical beauty.

In a comfortable seated position or in a chair, breathe out completely. Extend your tongue and curl the sides in, forming a tube shape (63). Breathe in slowly, then hold for a count of three. Exhale with mouth closed. Hold for a count of three. Make the inhalation and exhalation equal in length. Repeat 5 to 10 times.

Soft Bellows Breath *(Kapalabhati)*

This exercise tones and relaxes the muscles and nerves involved in respiration. It is an excellent preparatory technique for meditation because it focuses the mind very quickly. Its Sanskrit name literally means "shining skull," which refers to the power of this technique to stimulate the movement of energy through the body to the top of the head. In mythical language, this implies that a lotus is opening at the top of the head as the physical and emotional bodies become charged with energy from respiration.

Sit comfortably on the edge of a chair with feet tucked under slightly, or on the floor in a cross-legged position with your hips raised on cushions. You may rest one hand on your belly to monitor the movement, or rest your hands on your knees or thighs. In this exercise, you breathe in the same way as the Belly Breath but slightly faster so that you are moving the respiratory muscles a little more strongly. Breathe in for a count of three, then out for a count of three, without holding your breath either at the top or the bottom. The inhalation and exhalation should be equal in length. One cycle equals three inhalations and exhalations. Start with three cycles (nine breaths), and work up to 11 cycles (33 breaths). At the end of each cycle, relax your breath and rest for at least a count of three.

Chapter 5

Yoga Meditation for Arthritis

Your Meditation Position

In meditation you will be practicing "thinking nothing." To quiet your mind successfully, your physical body must be completely relaxed, and you cannot relax if you are straining to maintain an uncomfortable seated position. For this reason, we strongly suggest that you begin to learn meditation lying flat. That way, you can forget about your body while you focus on your thoughts and feelings. If your lower back feels tense, you can place a few pillows under your knees. Be careful to avoid pressure on the back of your neck. For this reason, it is best not to use a pillow; if you must have a pillow, it should be a small flat one.

If you are unable to lie on your back, you may sit in a chair as long as your back is straight — this is very important for meditation practice. Eventually, as you proceed in practice, you can try a comfortable seated position such as one of those described for the breathing exercises in Chapter 4 (see page 113).

Clothing and Equipment

Lie on the blanket or mat that you use for Yoga practice; if it is too short for your entire body, rest your head on it. Do not use a pillow under your head unless you have to, because it is important not to put pressure on the back of your neck. Wear your exercise clothes, and put on socks to keep your feet warm. Wrap your upper body with a shawl or blanket; your body temperature will drop as your body relaxes and your mind fills with silence, and you don't want to become chilled.

Protect Yourself from Disturbance

Ask family members not to interrupt you during your meditation time, and make sure pets are in another area. Turn off your telephone. Keep your practice space quiet and secure; sudden noises or intrusions can be quite shocking when you are completely relaxed and intensely quiet. Do not play music during any part of Yoga practice, because you want to experience your own thoughts and feelings free of outside influences. Silence is important.

Your Meditation Experience

Meditation is the key to bringing your two bodies, the physical and the emotional, together in harmony. If you practice a few minutes of meditation every day, along with a few exercises, it won't be long before you start to experience the satisfying power of operating as a whole person.

Meditation is not concentrating on your breath, or a sound, or anything else; it is simply no thought. One of the best ways to explain the meditation experience is that you simply try to stop talking to yourself. In the beginning, you may notice just a few seconds of quietness after you stop thinking one thought before another thought slips in. Meditation is a continuous process of increasing awareness. You start out in quietness, then before you know it your mind is full of plans, memories, anxieties, and other thoughts. Then you remember to stop talking to yourself, you are quiet for a while, and the whole process begins again. Try to remember what it feels like when you are not thinking. Eventually you will be able to re-create that feeling at will, and that will help you maintain the quiet feeling for longer periods of time.

Some people fall asleep when they first begin learning how to meditate. This is perfectly natural, and you will experience a very restful type of sleep. If you are practicing in the morning and are afraid that you will sleep too long, try not to use an alarm clock, because the loud noise will startle you and upset your system. Simply tell yourself mentally that you wish to meditate for a certain length of time and you will find that you naturally "wake up" after that time has passed. If you still need an aid to end meditation, try the alarm of a digital watch placed under a pillow so the sound is audible but not startling. I suggest that you begin by meditating for 10 minutes daily, and work up to 20 or 30 minutes if you wish.

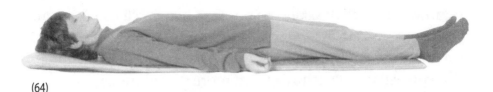

(64)

Complete Relaxation Procedure

Lie on your back with your arms at your sides, palms up. Let your fingers curl naturally, and let your feet fall slightly outward (64). This is called the Corpse Pose. This complete relaxation procedure will take 5 to 10 minutes. The idea is to completely relax every bone, muscle, and nerve in your body so that you can forget about your body while you meditate. An audiocassette of the entire relaxation/meditation procedure is available from the American Yoga Association; see Resources.

Read over the following directions and then close your eyes and begin relaxing. You will be focusing your attention quietly on each part of your body, visualizing each part in turn without moving any part of your body except your breath. Simply tell yourself to relax each body part in your mind.

Start with your face. Gently and calmly bring all of your attention to your forehead. Feel all of the muscles in your forehead. Let them relax so they feel loose.

Become aware of your eyes. Are they tense and jumpy? The eyes are usually the most difficult body part to relax, so just let them loosen and float in the sockets. Let all tension and movement in the eyes stop. Move on to your lips, teeth, and all the muscles of the jaw, mouth, and throat. Let your tongue relax in your mouth, and say to yourself, "I don't have to speak for a few minutes." Feel all the skin on your face become loose. Let your scalp relax and imagine your ears drooping toward the floor. Your eyes may continue to jump around a little, but after regular practice you will be able to relax them more and more.

Now relax your shoulders, arms, and hands. Feel as if your arms were hollow. Let all the muscles of the shoulders settle loosely on the floor. Move down into your elbow joints and imagine you can see and feel the bones. Relax and loosen them. Do the same with your forearms, wrists, and right into your hands and fingers, making them hollow and loose. Relax your fingers completely as though they were empty gloves lying on the floor.

Silently move your attention, like a tiny, warm relaxing beam of light, into your chest and, for a few moments, just observe the air moving in and out of your lungs. Feel your heart beating softly and rhythmically. Notice your belly rising and falling as you breathe. Do not try to speed up or slow down your breathing. Instead, just picture your lungs. Then take in a gentle breath of air, and, just as though you are sighing, let the breath out and relax your lungs. Take in another deep, gentle breath, sigh it out, and feel your heart relaxing also. Then let go of your breathing altogether, and relax all tension or effort in your breathing. Observe your belly and try to relax the squeezing effort as you breathe out. Each time you exhale, make your breath as relaxed as possible so that you are exerting almost no effort to breathe.

Now move your attention down into your legs, picturing them hollow, just as you did with your arms. Loosen and relax your thighs, hip sockets, and groin. Relax your knee joints and feel as though your lower legs are also hollow and empty, all the way into your toes. Imagine that your feet are empty — nothing inside, not even any bones. Feel your toenails relax and loosen.

Move up inside your empty feet, legs, and thighs, and bring your attention to the base of your spine. As you move upward through your waist area, relax any sign of tension so that your entire spine feels rubbery and loose. Feel your spine and all of its joints all the way up to the base of your skull. Spend a little extra time at the back of your neck. This common tension site needs extra attention. Imagine you can look right down inside your spinal column as though your spine were a rope dangling down into a dark well. Relax your spine so much that it feels as loose as that rope.

Next, concentrate on moving inside your head. Bring your attention back to your face to check whether or not your face is tense. Relax your eyes even more now, and let them float almost as though you can't feel them move at all.

Recheck the three main tension areas. 1) Is your breathing relaxed? 2) Are your eyes and facial muscles relaxed? 3) Is the back of your neck relaxed? Your body will eventually feel as if it were just an empty shell with no tension anywhere. The only movement will be your heart and your breathing, but they also will be very relaxed. Now relax the entire inside of your head. Feel your brain quietly settling inside your head with no effort or strain — just quiet and still.

Here is a summary of the relaxation steps:

1. *Relax your face and eyes.*

2. *Relax and empty your arms and hands.*

3. *Relax your lungs and heart.*

4. *Relax your belly and breathing.*

5. *Relax and empty your legs and feet, especially your thighs and knees.*

6. *Relax and loosen your back, shoulders, and neck.*

7. *Relax the inside of your head.*

8. *Recheck the three major tension areas: 1) your face and eyes; 2) your breathing; 3) the back of your neck.*

Meditation

Now you are ready to meditate. Start your meditation period by thinking of the sound "Om" (pronounced "ohm"). This word is a sound formula that has a specific effect on the mind when it is repeated or heard. "Om" is the oldest and most basic sound in classical Yoga. It has been said that if you could hear the subtle humming sound of the collective atomic structure of your own body and mind, that sound would most resemble the sound Om.

The Om sound of classical Yoga has been adopted and used in a religious way by nearly every religion of the Eastern world. However, in classical Yoga, the sound Om is used to center and focus the mind, and is not meant to indicate any particular religious concept or deity. Its purpose is to empty the mind except for the sound itself, leading finally to complete silence.

When you practice meditation, you will probably find that your experience of silence will be deeper and more refreshing if you repeat the sound "Om" to yourself several times at the beginning of your meditation session. Then simply stop talking to yourself in your mind. Try to stop all inner conversation. Don't force it; meditation is a process, not something that can be mastered overnight. Treat your daily meditation session like a game; see how long you can be still before a thought interrupts you. Some days you will be able to be still for a long time; other days it will be difficult to stop talking to yourself or stop thinking even for a second. Just keep trying every day and focus on the refreshing, quiet feeling that stays with you after your meditation session.

Eventually you will notice that this feeling will accompany you throughout your day. All you have to do is remember the feeling and it will be there. Many students tell me that their daily meditation period is as refreshing as taking a short nap. It is a tremendous help to concentration.

After Meditation

How you come out of meditation is as important as how you relax into it. If you get up too quickly, you may feel irritable or upset. When you open your eyes, before you start to move around, lie still for a few minutes longer thinking about the sensations, feelings, and thoughts that you experienced during your meditation period. Then increase your breathing a little to start reactivating your body and consciousness. At first, when you go to move your hands and arms, they may feel a little like wood since they've become so utterly relaxed. Make fists with your hands; then release them. Keeping your legs straight on the floor, flex your feet back toward your chin and then point them away. Do this a few times. Stretch your arms and legs like a cat does when it awakens from a nap. As you move toward your normal activities, you will feel refreshed, alert, and recharged with new energy and a clear mind.

Chapter 6

Yoga Fantasy Techniques for Arthritis

If you have arthritis, the constant worry about pain occupies a great part of your conscious and unconscious thoughts. It is always on your mind, and it affects all the decisions and relationships in your life. "Is the pain going to go away? Is it going to come back? Will I be able to do what I want to do today? I feel badly that I snapped at my spouse because I was in pain and just couldn't stand one more thing."

Those lucky few whose bodies never betray them with pain and suffering seldom understand the continual drain of personal power that such discomfort causes. A loss of confidence accompanies all your activities, as well as loss of a pleasing self-image. If you don't feel your best, you usually feel that you don't look your best, and seldom find the courage to compete in daily life activity. It takes a brave person to live a full life in spite of pain, and without becoming someone whose only conversation is complaint. Pain may be a constant; how it affects you depends on the support that you are able to elicit from your inner body. The self-confidence that brings this about can come from the practice of Yoga, particularly through the use of fantasy.

Fantasy will help you adjust to a new way of feeling as you progress with our program. The choice of what to talk about, for example, is sometimes a shock, because spending months or years talking mostly about pain is now a lot less true about your life as the pain itself recedes and, at the same time, you learn different ways to cope. The physical body invents clever ways to keep its attitude from changing; you can counteract that tendency by trying to see yourself in a new body — one that is supple, relaxed, healthy, beautiful, and pain-free — each day in fantasy.

Many times, self-destructive attitudes are hidden in our vision of ourselves. Constant effort must be made to change your vision of yourself to what you want it to be, not a vision that portrays you as a victim. I have observed that most physical pain and stiffness is due to one or the other of our bodies, the spiritual or the physical, acting with vengeance on the other. Imagine yourself looking into a mirror and saying "I hate my body for feeling so crippled!" Imagine your physical body feeling fear and upset because of impending attack, and the emotional/spiritual body saying, "Wait a minute here, this is my production and don't fool with it!" This is not a peaceful place to play! Our game becomes a reality when we then punish ourselves with unhealthy food, alcohol, or drugs, whipping ourselves with violent practices that throw us out of harmony and balance.

Often, in their zeal to begin getting results, people rush into a harsh discipline that upsets both bodies, setting the stage for the kind of vengeful reactions described previously. I suggest that you do not force a quick and ruthless change of attitudes upon yourself. Start slowly, and create a gradual change of lifestyle that allows your physical and emotional bodies to get used to the new routine, making it much more likely that you will continue. Most importantly, every day practice a fantasy vision of yourself as you wish to be. This is the key to establishing that new vision as you continue to change your behavior.

How to Practice Fantasy Exercises

In the following pages I will teach you some easy Fantasy techniques to practice as part of your daily Yoga routine. The first time you practice a Fantasy exercise, set aside 10 to 15 minutes in a private place where you won't be disturbed. After you are familiar with the techniques, you can try practicing them while walking (see Chapter 7), or you can incorporate them into many other activities of daily life. An excellent time to practice Fantasy is just before you go to sleep at night. Note: Please do not practice Fantasy exercises while driving, operating dangerous machinery, or any other activity that requires your full attention for safety reasons. Consider your focus on safety at those times to be a practice of the Yogic ethic of Nonviolence toward yourself, and remember to practice your Fantasy exercises at another time.

Creating a Vision of Yourself

Start by looking at yourself in a mirror, preferably full-length. Look at yourself for a minute or two, reminding yourself of all the things that you have said to yourself before about what you like or do not like about yourself, and how you feel about the different parts of your body, particularly the joints that erupt in pain or discomfort. Now sit or lie down in a comfortable position and close your eyes. Take a few deep Complete Breaths and then let your breath return to normal. Let your entire body go limp and relaxed. In your mind, imagine yourself standing in front of the mirror again, but this time, visualize yourself the way you would like to be. If your goal is to loosen and relax your joints, picture yourself with supple, graceful limbs, with no swollen or distorted joints. If you are also working on posture and muscle tone, picture yourself standing straight and proud. Don't limit yourself to physical attributes; picture yourself confident, poised, radiant with good health and strength — every desirable quality that you can think of. Hold that vision in your mind for as long as you can in silence. Then take another deep breath, let it out, and notice how you feel. Tell yourself how you feel, and remind yourself that you can recall that feeling whenever you need it or want it. Open your eyes and go about your day with new energy.

The "I Love You" Meditation Technique

Throughout this book, I talk about the importance of self-confidence in the management of arthritis. This technique is one of the best ways I know to give yourself the confidence you need and want. It is easy to do, and once you learn the technique, I urge you to use it throughout the day in different ways. For example, one of my students stands in front of the mirror every morning drying his hair. All the time his blow-dryer is on, he repeats "I love you" to his reflection in the mirror until his hair is dry. He says that this simple practice has changed his life.

This technique is a complement to, not a substitute for, daily meditation practice. (An audiocassette of this technique is available from the American Yoga Association; see Resources.) You will need to set aside about 15 to 20 minutes for this technique. Try it just before bed for a restful, refreshing sleep. Prepare yourself just as if you were going into meditation: lie on your back on your blanket, keep warm, and protect yourself from disturbances.

Start with what may seem a strange technique: Pump your arms and legs vigorously as if you were riding a bicycle, so that your whole body is moving. Laugh out loud and be as silly as you can imagine for about 30 seconds! This exercise will stimulate the brain chemicals that contribute to feelings of well-being. Then relax your body, settle in to your meditation position, and let your breath relax.

Bring your attention to your forehead. Breathe in, saying "I love you" to yourself. Do the same as you breathe out. Repeat several times: breathe in "I love you" and breathe out "I love you." Breathe in and hold for a moment. Imagine the feeling "I love you" spreading throughout your brain in a beautiful, warm, wet, perfumed essence. Breathe out "I love you."

Relax completely. Let your breath relax. Hold that feeling. Then, for a few more minutes, continue saying "I love you" each time you breathe in and out. As you breathe in and hold your breath for a moment, think to yourself, "Whom do I love?" Breathe out and say "I love you." Breathe in and hold again; think: "Who loves me?" Now think to yourself: "My breath loves me." Breathe out. "My breath loves me." The breath is inside you. It loves you. Breathe in and think "I'm holding my breath — it loves me." Breathe out and think "I have released my breath — it still loves me." Take a deep breath, always through your nose. Breathe in: "My breath loves me." Breathe out: "My breath is gone now but it still loves me."

Relax completely. Visualize the inside of your head and your body. Think of the breath commingled with love. Oxygen is flowing through your arteries and heart and every part of you because you can't live without your breath. Visualize this loving breath inside your body. Are there any blocks keeping it from moving where it wants to go? Visualize this feeling of love and breath removing any kind of constriction, moving easily and sweetly throughout your body.

Bring the feeling to your forehead. Think "I love you — my breath is in my forehead." Relax your forehead. Now think of this feeling of love spreading to your eyes — you can almost see it! Relax your eyes and let the breath of love simply swim out into the rest of your face. Feel this breath of love in your nose, because it breathes for you. Every time you breathe in, breathe "I love you." Every time you breathe out, breathe "I love you." Let the breath of love flow freely so that your face melts with love. Let your mouth and throat relax, thinking "I love you" as you breathe.

Let your neck relax now so you have no constriction that will stop the breath from moving. Love comes in with your breath — relax. Love goes out with your breath — relax. Drop your collarbone toward the floor and say "I love you." Let the ends of your shoulders drop. Do the same with your arms; let them relax; feel that they are fully supported by this breath of love. Rest your arms in love. Relax your wrists. Let your hands be totally relaxed in love. You're vulnerable. You don't care. You can't lose love. Breath comes in and it goes out, and love is still there. Relax your fingers, letting them curl slightly, like a baby's hand when it is asleep.

Move your attention to your chest. Be aware that you are taking a breath into your heart: "I love you." Breathe it out with love. Breathe into your lungs: "I love you." Breathe out "I love you." Now relax your entire chest. Let your breath relax in love. Become aware that this breath is love. You're not making it happen; it's happening because it loves you.

Breathe in and think of your stomach. Breathe out and say "I love you" as you relax your stomach. Relax your abdomen, thinking: "I love you. I love you the way you are." Feel the breath of love move through your hip joints. Warm, liquid, lubricating, beautiful — perfectly balanced and poised. Say "I love you" to your hips and relax them. Let the large bones in the top of your legs sink toward the floor; you don't have to hold them up. You love them. They love you. You can't lose love. Relax your legs in love. Relax your knees and ankles and think "I love you." Think to your feet "I love you." Relax your feet.

Picture yourself just simply floating; completely supported on this breath, this love. Bring your attention up to the back of your hips and the base of your spine. Open it up like a flower. Say "I love you." Don't fight it. Let it flow easily, smooth and quiet. Relax the back of your shoulder blades. Let your back get soft. Love is supporting you. "I love you, back." The back of your neck relaxes. Think to yourself, "I love you. I love you." Then you reach your brain, your hair, all soft and supported, resting in love, in breath.

Breathe in and think love. Breathe out — love is still there. Think of your brain floating in a pool of this love. Make it totally quiet. Then simply say to yourself, "I love you." Bring your mind to your forehead and think nothing. Hold this feeling of quietness. If you feel any other thought coming in, make sure that it says "I love you." Transpose any thought to "I love you" and go back to thinking nothing. Think nothing as long as you can. Stop talking to yourself. Become silent internally.

Rest quietly like this for about ten minutes, then slowly stretch, take a deep breath and let it out, and think about how you feel. Rest on your side or stomach for a few minutes enjoying the feeling before you get up. Move slowly back into your normal attitudes and lifestyle with a new vision of yourself.

During this exercise, it is important to note who is loving you. Regular practice of the "I love you" technique will open expression channels for your inner emotional body. It gives attention to the body that will replace the tension and stiffness that accompany pain. Every time you take something away from the physical body it must be offered a replacement for what it has lost or it will take vengeance on the emotional body. Similarly, if you deny expression to the emotional body, it will take vengeance on the physical. The goal is to find a happy balance where neither body fears the other. Fantasy is the best way to achieve this balance, and the "I love you" technique is the basis for this practice of providing daily attention to the body in other ways than acknowledging suffering.

The Hall of Doors

This technique is very helpful for concentrating on a particular problem or concern. For example, suppose interaction with a particular person is so stressful that your joints always become tense and painful after you see this person. Using this technique, you can practice those stressful interactions and perhaps change the way you respond. Another example is fear of failure, something that nearly everyone who begins a new exercise program faces in some measure. This technique will help you face your fear and build the strength to overcome it.

This fantasy exercise requires a concentrated period of about 5 to 10 minutes. Lie down on your back on your mat in the Corpse Pose with your arms at your sides, legs together, and eyes closed. Don't use a pillow behind your head. You can also do this exercise sitting in a chair as long as your back is straight. Stay warm. Completely relax your body as if you were about to meditate (see page 123).

Begin your fantasy exercise by bringing your inner attention to your forehead. Imagine that you are looking down a long hallway. There are several doors leading off this central hallway — some to the left, some to the right. Picture the hallway in every detail: the color of the walls, whether the floor is carpet, tile, or wood; the color of and type of hardware on the doors; the lighting in the hallway — invent all these small details in your fantasy. Make it complete in your mind before you enter it.

Now before you walk down the hall, protect yourself by covering your entire body with armor. Imagine the most beautiful, heroic suit that you can, with all of the details, such as the color and weight of the armor, the type of helmet and gloves, the boots, and the fastenings. When your body is completely protected with armor, then create a beautiful sword of your own design and take it in your hand.

The reason for all this protection is that, in fantasy, you are exploring the unknown realm of your unconscious. Although everything in your mind is part of you, much of it will seem unfamiliar, and it might even feel a bit frightening at first. Our conscious mind often feels anxiety about anything that is unknown; the symbolic protection of the armor and sword that you create in your mind lets you enter and observe your fantasy world without fear.

When you have a clear picture of your armor and sword, imagine yourself entering the hallway. Each door has the name of some problem or concern written on it. Choose one of the doors, put your hand on the knob, and open it. Stand protected by your armor and sword, and simply observe what is in that room. Realize that you can step back and shut the door anytime you wish. I suggest that at first you try to observe for about a minute before leaving the room. When you decide to leave, shut the door, walk back down the hall, remove your armor, and observe yourself resting in the Corpse Pose. Give yourself plenty of time to change your orientation from the fantasy experience back to resting. Then, for a few minutes, think about what you have discovered.

The names on the various doors in your hallway can correspond to the concerns that are uppermost in your mind as you work with your arthritis management program. Some examples are fear of movement, self-hate, pain, anxiety about your ability to function normally, difficulty in a relationship, pressure at work, and so on. Do not try to open all the doorways in one session; one at a time is enough! Try a new one each week.

Sometimes students tell me that they feel like quitting in frustration, saying that they never see anything when they open the doors in their fantasy. Usually I find that these people are afraid to try, which tells me that the obstacle confronting them is very difficult. If you find yourself in this position, simply continue with the fantasy exercise until you begin to enjoy some success. Probably you have never attempted to communicate with your unconscious mind before. If you continue to do the technique, eventually something will appear. I have never known a student who didn't eventually find something behind a door.

This technique will work best if you can practice it daily for at least a week. You will quickly experience great improvement in your concentration and your ability to deal with daily problems. Most of all, however, regular practice of this exercise allows the hidden, unseen experience of your inner body to show itself to you. It is no longer something that you just feel; it takes shape, and you are fully protected to face it and respond to it. When you have mastered the technique, you will find that you can use it as an immediate solution to whatever problems are hindering your progress in your arthritis management program.

Chapter 7

Walking Contemplation for Arthritis

When you are coping with arthritis, regular exercise is important. Exercise burns calories, helping you to lose weight that puts extra stress on your joints. Exercise also helps to reduce pain and stiffness, by keeping joints flexible and circulation strong. Regular exercise feels good, too. When you are active, your body circulates more blood to your brain, bringing it more oxygen and releasing the chemicals called endorphins that contribute to feelings of well-being.

In this chapter, I am going to teach you how to incorporate regular exercise into your daily life as part of your Yoga routine for arthritis. If you can get into the habit of doing your Yoga routine every day, you will improve your concentration and your health, and you will enjoy exercise more. It won't become boring. Most importantly, you will feel less discomfort with everyday activities.

You can practice this technique while walking, swimming, or riding a stationary bicycle. I have chosen to focus on these three forms of exercise because they are easy to do and, more importantly, they are not dangerous to do while your attention is elsewhere. Walking and cycling also are quite effective at changing your metabolic rate. They are low-impact — much easier on your joints than running or other high-impact sports. I do not recommend cycling on the street, simply because you will have to pay too much attention to traffic and other hazards to be able to concentrate fully on the technique. If you are an experienced exerciser used to running or jogging, you can try adapting this technique for use on a treadmill.

Bhairavi Mudra

This technique, which I am calling "walking contemplation," is based on an ancient Yogic technique called *Bhairavi Mudra* (bye-RAH-vee MOO-dra). Both of my great teachers used to use this technique while walking in the mountains of Kashmir. Here is a rough translation of the verse that describes the technique:

> *Bhairavi Mudra is a pose in which the eyes are open externally without blinking, but the attention is turned to the inner essential Self. Though the eyes are open, the aspirant sees nothing of the external world.*

This is a bit like meditating with your eyes open. Think of the "inner essential Self" as the feeling of stillness that you experience while meditating (see Chapter 5). While you are walking (or swimming or cycling), simply turn your mind inward and try to reexperience the feeling of stillness. Stop talking to yourself internally.

Try to turn all your senses inward as well. For instance, you see the roses in your neighbor's garden as you pass by. While practicing Walking Contemplation, you try not to name the flowers or let your thoughts turn to your own garden; you just experience the sensation of seeing the colors and shapes and move on as you feel stillness inside. You may hear birds singing, or other noises; try not to name the noise or look for it, but simply walk on with your attention turned to inner silence. In other words, try not to use language in the experience.

You will find this to be a continual process. Just as in the concentrated meditation period that you do as part of your daily Yoga routine (see Chapter 7), you will find that sometimes it is easier to feel stillness than at other times. In the beginning, you may be able to focus on stillness only for a few seconds at a time. Eventually, something that you see or hear or remember starts the thinking — and inner talking — again. Whenever you notice yourself thinking about something else, gently bring your attention back to stillness. Don't force it, and try not to judge yourself. Look at it like a game that you are playing with yourself. See how long you can do it.

When I first began this practice, I tried it while walking through a department store and was overwhelmed by the seemingly infinite number of recognitions, categorizations, and even judgments that my brain was capable of producing. It was as if the

The Ethic of Nonhoarding

The practice of Bhairavi Mudra will sharpen your awareness of the subtle aspects of hoarding. Whenever you name an object that you see — flowers, fence, etc. — you are, in a sense, owning that object. In Walking Contemplation, you are trying to reduce that outward reach of your mind in order to focus on the feeling of stillness. The experience of that stillness, where "names and forms" (*namarupa*, in Sanskrit) leave the mind, is one aspect of the ethical practice of Nonhoarding.

huge number of objects surrounding me were all demanding a response from me, which was distracting and upsetting, even to the point of often making me sick to my stomach. If you find that you are always tired after a shopping trip, perhaps you are experiencing this also, and you might find the technique of Bhairavi Mudra helpful. After long practice of this technique myself, I have found that the chaos of these earlier adventures is much reduced, and trips to the mall are a lot more peaceful.

If you find that it is too hard to focus on stillness at first, or if you just want a change of pace, you can substitute other subjects for contemplation. Here are a few suggestions:

Focus on Nonviolence, or some other ethic. Use your exercise time to consider how you can practice Nonviolence in yourself, such as stopping self-critical thoughts, counteracting feelings of helplessness, eating the right foods, and so on. (If you are interested in finding out more about Nonviolence and other ethics of Yoga, they are discussed at length in my book *Yoga of the Heart*; see Resources.)

In other sessions, focus on practicing Nonviolence toward others, such as a spouse, child, or co-worker; think about some ways in which you may have acted in a hurtful way toward the person, and mentally rehearse future interactions in which you respond nonviolently.

Practice the "I Love you" technique. While you are exercising, practice the "I Love You" technique in your mind (see page 131), repeating the phrase on your breath and carrying it throughout your body just as if you were lying down.

Watch your breath. In the same way that you concentrate on stillness, concentrate on your breath. Do not change your breath; simply watch it. Listen to the sound of your breath as you walk. (See page 113 for more on the sound of your breath.) It helps to talk to your breath: Encourage it and praise it.

Beginning Your Exercise Program

Following are some tips to make the exercise portion of this technique more effective. Although these instructions focus primarily on walking, you can easily adapt them for swimming and cycling. I've added some particular recommendations for each form of exercise.

Start Gradually

The most common mistake people make in beginning a new exercise program is overdoing it, demanding too much of muscles that are not accustomed to being worked and creating stress by making too drastic a lifestyle change all at once. By gradually incorporating small increments of exercise time into your daily schedule, you will start looking forward to the feelings of relaxation and stress relief that exercise brings rather than seeing it as "one more thing I have to do today." If you start slowly, and gradually build up your exercise time, you will be more likely to enjoy it and keep it up as part of your new healthy lifestyle.

I find that people often overdo in the beginning, not out of naïve overenthusiasm but actually in order to defeat the effort. As I discussed in previous chapters, if the inner emotional body is not acknowledged and nourished, it will do everything it can to return the body to its previous state. The inner emotional body sabotages our plans with an initial euphoria which urges us to do more than we can sustain, making it more likely that we will overdo and eventually quit altogether. If you notice this tendency in yourself, try to restrain the impulse to do too much, and reassure your inner body with statements such as "Little by little, I am changing my vision of myself. I will love the way I look and feel as I gradually create new enjoyable habits of diet and exercise." Another way to acknowledge your inner body is through fantasy: Try the fantasy exercise of the Hall of Doors, picture your frightened inner body in one of the rooms, and then console it, "sweet-talk" it, and develop a closer communication with it.

Whether you are a very sedentary person who is unaccustomed to any exercise, or someone who is more active and wants to adopt a more regular fitness program, we recommend this single goal for the first two weeks: Get out the door and walk (or swim, or cycle) for a comfortable period of time four times each week. Don't worry about time, mileage, or pacing; simply get used to practicing the contemplation exercise while you are exercising. It may be 5 minutes, it may be 20 minutes; just enjoy the benefits of taking care of yourself. Give your body a chance to enjoy a little exercise without taking the approach of a stern taskmaster. Schedule your exercise session when pain and stiffness are at a minimum.

Keep in mind that the goal is to develop a new lifestyle; a new way of looking at what is important to health and well-being each day. Although we recommend exercising four days per week in the beginning, set your goal on attaining at least five days of exercise per week eventually, and preferably seven days. If you start slowly and progress gradually, you will enjoy exercising so much that you won't want to miss a day!

Beginning in week three, add five minutes to your exercise time each week (never add more than five minutes per week). In week four, take five minutes to warm up as part of your allotted time, pick up the pace a little during your main exercise period, then add five minutes for cool-down (see below). Continue adding five minutes per week until you reach a total of 40 minutes (5 minutes warm-up, 30 minutes brisk activity, 5 minutes cooldown) four or more days per week. See Resources for some excellent books on walking, cycling, and swimming if you'd like to refine your technique or add to your program.

Warm Up

Always begin your exercise session by walking slowly for 5 to 10 minutes to warm up your body before you begin exercising more vigorously. During that 5- to 10-minute warm-up, rotate your arms, shoulders, and head gently to loosen your upper

Incremental Exercise Works Too

You don't have to exercise all at once to reap the benefits of exercise. As long as the exercise is vigorous, you can achieve the same results in three 10-minute segments throughout the day as in 30 minutes of sustained exercise. You can also add even more exercise time to your day by doing such things as:

– parking at the far end of the lot and walking briskly into the store or work.

– taking the stairs instead of the elevator.

– walking the dog at a good pace.

Just remember that your total time spent in briskly paced activities each day should add up to at least 30 minutes (not counting warm-up and cool-down time).

body. If you are quite stiff, you may wish to do a few more range-of-motion exercises; see the warm-up section of Chapter 3 (pp. 53-79).

If you are cycling or swimming, do a few Arm Circles (p. 55) and Shoulder Rolls (p. 53) first, then ride or swim for a few minutes at a leisurely pace; in swimming, use a stroke that you enjoy most. If you are walking or riding a stationary bicycle, you will know that you are warmed up when you just begin to break a sweat.

Your Main Exercise Session

Adding no more than five minutes per week, work up to 30 minutes of continuous exercise at least four days per week, practicing the contemplation exercise each time. You should be walking (or riding, or swimming) hard enough so that you are breathing a little faster than usual, but not hard enough so you get winded.

Hints for walkers: Watch your posture: relax your shoulders, keep your chin down, and don't arch your lower back. Breathe through your nose at all times. Pumping your arms as you walk increases the aerobic benefit while building and toning muscles in the arms, shoulders, and upper and lower back. Bend elbows at a 90° angle, and loosely clench your fists. Move your arms straight forward and back, brushing the sides of your body. Though it may seem natural to let your arms cross toward the center of your body in the front, pumping straight forward and back requires more muscular control, is gentler on the shoulder joints, and helps to prevent low back pain.

Hints for swimmers: Use a variety of strokes: crawl/freestyle, breaststroke, sidestroke, backstroke. If you get winded, stop and tread water for a minute or two, or move to the side of the pool and practice some kicks (but try to maintain your contemplation exercise). Most authorities recommend continuing to move in some way during a recovery period rather than stopping completely. As your lung capacity improves, you'll be able to swim for longer periods. Note: there is some evidence that swimming is not as effective as dry-land exercise for losing body fat, because the water buoys you up and your muscles don't have to work as hard. Also, the cooling effect of the water means that your heart works less hard to do the same job. However, if you are new to exercise, swimming is a gentle, effective way to get into the exercise habit, and it is much gentler on the joints than dry-land exercise, making it a perfect way for arthritics to enjoy gentle exercise. You can also swim a few days per week, and walk or cycle other days. See the paragraph on "cross training," below.

Hints for cyclists: Your knees take less stress when you spin at a low gear (turning the cranks quickly and easily) instead of pushing a high gear (turning cranks slowly and with great effort). The combination of lower gear and fast cadence allows your muscles to work most efficiently. A long, steady ride trains your metabolism to burn fat more readily. If you are just starting out, take the time to choose a bicycle that fits correctly, and wear proper gear so that you remain comfortable. Find a location in your home where you can practice your contemplation exercise while riding, without becoming distracted by other family members, the television or radio, and so on.

Cross Training

Experienced athletes use cross training to increase their fitness and prevent injury. In cross training, you alternate two or, at the most, three forms of exercise during the week. Doing just one form of exercise trains only one set of muscles, while cross training works on different sets of muscles. For instance, cycling exercises the lower body primarily, while swimming adds emphasis to the upper body. Swimming may not burn fat as fast as walking because it is not a weight-bearing exercise; however, walking is harder on the joints, especially the knees, and can be more strenuous for some people, especially if you are extremely sedentary. Doing a small amount of two forms of exercise prevents injury by varying the work that your joints and muscles are required to do. And of course, preventing injury means no lost time from daily exercise. This technique also helps prevent boredom in your routine.

Wind Sprints (Interval Training)

A wind sprint is a short burst of higher intensity exercise in the middle of low-intensity exercise. For instance, after walking at your normal pace for 5 to 10 minutes, speed up to a much faster walk for 20 to 60 seconds, then slow back to your regular pace. Repeat every 5 to 10 minutes during your walking session. You can do the same while swimming or cycling. This short burst adds intensity to your exercise session without risking injury, and the brief extra work on your muscles means a more efficient fat-burning effect overall.

Cool Down

The cool-down period is as important as the warm-up. Walk, swim, or cycle at a slow pace for 5 to 10 minutes, then do a few stretches (on land) to lengthen the muscles that have contracted while you were exercising. If you don't stretch, your muscles will continue to contract and eventually start hurting due to the build-up of lactic acid. Here are some easy stretches that will work for either walking, swimming, or cycling:

Calf and Achilles' tendon stretches: (1) Stand facing a wall and rest your hands on the wall. Stand with back straight and abdominals in. Place right foot forward about six inches from the wall, and left foot back. Both heels remain flat on the floor, toes pointing forward. Ease your pelvis forward to feel the stretch in the main body of your left calf. Hold 10 to 15 seconds, then switch sides.

(2) Placing hands on the wall as before, stand with feet together about two feet away from the wall, toes forward and heels down. Keeping hips tucked in, gently bend knees until you feel the stretch in your lower calf and Achilles' tendon. Hold 10 to 15 seconds.

Toe Points and Ankle Circles: Holding on to a chair or bench for balance, straighten one leg in front of you and point your toes, then flex them. Repeat several times, then switch legs. Next, stretch one leg in front of you and rotate the ankle 5 to 10 times in each direction. Repeat with the other ankle.

Forward Bend: Stand with feet parallel, a few inches apart. Breathe in deeply, stretching your arms wide to the sides, then breathe out and bend forward, keeping your knees straight but not locked (if you have any lower back discomfort, you can bend your knees slightly). Let your upper body relax, especially your arms and head. Stay in the forward position for about 20 seconds, breathing normally. Then breathe in as you slowly straighten.

Heel Back: Holding on to a chair or bench for balance with your left hand, bend your right knee and grasp the toes of your right foot with your right hand. Pull the foot gently toward your body, stopping when you feel a pull in your thigh. Hold for about 20 seconds, breathing normally. Do this twice on each leg, alternating.

Shoulder Stretch: Reach straight up with one hand as if trying to touch the ceiling. Now reach up behind your head with the other hand and pull the elbow across above your head slowly.

Stop as soon as you feel a gentle pull in the shoulder, armpit, or back. Hold for a count of 20, breathing normally, then slowly release and relax. Do this twice on each side, alternating.

Chapter 8

Diet and Nutrition for Arthitis

I recommend a diet for arthritis that is adequate in all nutrients, with a goal of achieving and/or maintaining your ideal weight. This basic diet plan is rich in fruits and vegetables, high in carbohydrates, and low in fat. It is also rich in antioxidants, such as vitamins C and E, beta-carotene, and selenium to help protect the cartilage and facilitate the repair/rebuilding process.

I recommend that everyone with arthritis try glucosamine and chondroitin for at least three months to find out if it benefits them. Please see the following chapter for more information. Any of these alternatives should be tried for three months minimum and then discarded if not effective for you. Remember that no supplement can substitute for a balanced diet; the basic diet described in this chapter, rich in fresh fruits and vegetables and low in fat, with the right amount of vitamins and minerals, will always be beneficial.

The Yoga arthritis diet is grounded in the idea of Nonviolence, the first and foremost of the ethical guidelines that are the basis of Yoga philosophy. When most people think about this ethic, they think of not harming others, but in Yoga practice your first duty is to not harm yourself. The strength of the partnership between your physical and spiritual bodies depends upon an attitude of help, not harm. Eating well is the most important act of kindness you can give to your physical body.

Arthritis and Overweight

After Nonviolence, the most important topic concerning diet and arthritis is achieving and/or maintaining your ideal weight. As I discussed in Chapter 2, overweight is a major risk factor in osteoarthritis, especially for hips and knees; the extra weight is suspected to increase the load and pressure on these weight-bearing joints. Even more importantly, losing weight has been shown to relieve osteoarthritis symptoms such as pain and stiffness.

But there is more to it than this, as overweight people also have a higher risk of osteoarthritis of the hands, suggesting that some metabolic factor is at work affecting joints not directly involved with bearing weight. It could well be more than an unfortunate coincidence that exactly the same population most prone to overweight is also most at risk for osteoarthritis: older women and men. Excess weight is well known to increase the risk of high blood pressure, heart disease, strokes, some cancers, and diabetes. Being overweight can also hurt your inner self: Depression, anxiety, and low self-esteem can result from excess weight gain. This makes it essential to find a way to maintain (or achieve) a normal weight in a healthy way that is also satisfying enough to your inner body that you can continue your new eating and activity habits indefinitely; in other words, to permanently change your lifestyle. Our arthritis program is all about permanently changing the way you eat, breathe, exercise — even the way you relax!

Achieving and maintaining normal weight is a good way to begin practicing Nonviolence toward yourself. By adding generous amounts of beneficial joint-protecting and -rebuilding foods and supplements, you have a much better chance of increasing mobility, and thus quality of life. I recommend that you do this by balancing diet and physical activity, resulting in health and strength while losing weight safely. In this chapter, I will present a detailed outline of how to change your eating habits so that you can supply the raw materials to protect and rebuild your joints. The Yogic approach to arthritis and diet is a lifestyle change that will help you all your life.

Some Tips on How to Lose Weight

1. Try to become more aware of how you feel when you eat by trying the Wrist Tape technique (see page 41 for full instructions). This technique has helped many of my students when they are trying to become more aware of some particular behavior. Place a piece of nonirritating tape (first-aid adhesive tape, painter's masking tape, or a simple Band-Aid works well) on your wrist every day for one week. Whenever you eat something, write "F" on the tape if you are eating because you need fuel, "B" if you are eating because you are bored, or "S" if you are stressed. At the end of the week, add up the three categories to show you how your mood affects how you eat. If you often eat when bored or stressed, that should indicate to you that it is important to find some substitute activities to nourish and care for your emo-

tional needs; otherwise, it will be much harder to lose weight. Make a list of other things to do instead of eating and post it where it will do the most good: on the fridge!

2. Follow the old saying, "Eat breakfast like a king, lunch like a prince, and supper like a pauper." It really does make a difference when you eat, because calories consumed when you are inactive — which for most people is at the end of the day — are more likely to be stored as fat. Fuel up before the most active part of your day and you will also be less likely to "diet" all day and "blow it" at night.

3. Learn your caloric needs (see Resources for some good books and other help) for simply maintaining your current weight. Subtract 500 calories daily to lose a pound per week. The calories saved can also come from increased aerobic activity: you can figure about 300 calories are burned per one hour of moderately paced exercise such as brisk walking (see Chapter 7 for our walking program).

4. Eat meals sitting down, and pace your eating, because it takes at least 20 minutes for the food to enter your bloodstream, sending a signal to your brain that you've had enough. Eat slowly and enjoy your meal. It is often a good idea to start with a low-calorie salad or a broth-type soup to make the meal last longer and fill you up sooner.

5. Do not try to deprive yourself of your favorite foods. The most likely outcome of dieting in my experience is "reward bingeing," where we say to ourselves, "I've been good all day, now I deserve that jelly doughnut (or a double date — you know, the one with Ben and Jerry!"). Enjoy your favorite food once a week: look forward to it, enjoy it, savor each yummy, greasy creamy bite! — and then move on.

6. Use the Yoga Fantasy techniques (see Chapter 6) to build a picture of yourself as you want to be: thinner, lighter, filled with health, free from pain, and so on. Start your day by filling your mind with positive visions of yourself to counteract feelings of failure and frustration that are actually violent toward yourself.

7. Keep in mind that when you eat well without abusing your physical body with food, you will feel better, have more energy to exercise and engage in activities that you love, and take the biggest step you can toward reducing the pain and stiffness of arthritis.

Despite what the popular magazines try to tell you, there is no magic pill or instant-success system for either curing arthritis or losing weight. There is no getting around the simple fact that to lose weight you must eat fewer calories than you burn up in physical activity. This of course becomes more difficult when arthritis reduces mobility, and when pain and stiffness discourage calorie-burning exercise. The same exercises that help arthritis are also good for calorie burning. The easiest and healthiest way to burn more calories consistently is to exercise regularly and reduce your intake of the nonessential calories from the "calorie-dense" foods: those high in fat and/or sugar. This leaves you with plenty of nutritious foods to eat that not only build health, but also satisfy your hunger. I'll give you some specific examples later in the chapter.

It is essential to increase your activity level by following the routines outlined in this book; a nutritious diet cannot provide enough essential nutrients and still be low enough in calories for your body to burn fat if you are inactive. When you are inactive, your muscles start wasting away, and your percentage of body fat soars. Muscle cells use calories faster than fat cells, so you would have to restrict your calorie intake even more just to

·maintain weight, much less lose extra pounds. It is also important to remember that metabolism naturally slows down with
age, so a constant activity level is necessary to counteract these
additional effects. The Yoga exercises presented in Chapter 3 help
to maintain the most efficient metabolism; they are easy enough
that they can be done every day, and many can be adapted for
practice in a chair or even in bed, so the benefits can continue
despite injury, illness, or age.

Arthritis and Essential Nutrients

The best way to control weight and keep your joints healthy is
to learn what nutrients are required for joint health and how to
create a diet that contains them in concentrated form, without
adding unnecessary calories from nonessential fats and sugars.

The Role of Antioxidants

Some specific relationships between nutrients and health are
well known. For instance, vitamin C levels are reduced in the
joint fluid and blood of rheumatoid arthritis patients, so some
experts have speculated that vitamin C supplementation would
benefit rheumatoid symptoms. However, there is as yet no con-
vincing evidence that vitamin C is therapeutic. Vitamins D, C,
and E are all vital for cartilage repair, so if they are adequately
supplied, osteoarthritis progression can be slowed, or even prevented or postponed. In many studies, researchers have noticed
that those with higher intakes of these nutrients show the beginning signs of osteoarthritis, but the joint degeneration is
stopped. In other words, the joint cartilage does not continue to
break down.

Another reason that vitamins C and E are important is because recent research has shown that certain joint cells are potent sources of oxidants that can damage cartilage and other joint tissue. Dietary antioxidants are your body's best defense against this type of damage, and thus may play an important role in slowing, postponing, or preventing osteoarthritis. Selenium and beta-carotene are other important antioxidants. One study did show that a history of higher intakes of vitamin C was associated with a threefold reduction in osteoarthritis of the knee. In another study, both lower blood levels and reduced dietary intake of vitamin D were associated with a three-fold increased risk for both knee and hip osteoarthritis.

Optimum nutrition, especially from antioxidants and vitamin D, seems to play a large role in preventing the pain and disability of osteoarthritis. Our Yoga diet plan includes lots of fresh fruits and vegetables that provide food-based antioxidants; vitamin D is added to many common foods, especially dairy, and is also formed on the skin by sunlight. In addition, our diet plan includes safe and effective supplements of all these vital nutrients. Vitamin D, by the way, is one of the handful of nutrients that can be toxic at high levels, so it is best to limit intake from all sources to no more than 400 IU daily.

Boron is a plentiful mineral found in many fruits and vegetables, nuts, and dried beans, and it has an important role in joint health, helping with calcium and magnesium metabolism. It serves as an antioxidant as well, and some evidence indicates that boron supplements can help ease the symptoms of both rheumatoid arthritis and osteoarthritis. Most experts agree that eating more fresh fruits and vegetables is the best way to get adequate boron; if supplements are used, limit intake to less than 3 mg daily.

Protein

The average American diet supplies about twice as much protein as is needed — usually accompanied by very nonessential saturated fat. Protein is required for building and repairing joint tissue, and for hormone production. Protein seems to play the primary role in the brain in reducing the hunger sensation, so adequate protein will help reduce cravings and hunger pangs, an important quality when you are trying to shed extra pounds to ease arthritis symptoms. However, excess protein usually adds a lot of unwanted calories and creates metabolic excess which the liver and kidneys must process and excrete.

On a low-calorie diet, the body may "panic," believing that it is starving. It then sets its metabolic rate lower in order to conserve energy, which prevents weight loss. To avoid this, be sure that protein is adequate in your diet. Protein should constitute about 15% of your caloric intake. If you follow the suggested diet plan in this chapter and obtain all the required servings of protein each day, you will be getting adequate protein. (A chart of protein needs is supplied in Chapter 9.)

Pure protein tablets provide as much as 1.9 grams of high-grade natural dairy protein per tablet. Since the tablets are pure protein, this source is the most efficient at delivering the maximum amount of protein for the lowest amount of calories. Plus, they are easily portable, so you can maintain your weight management diet in restaurants and at work or play. When using a pure source such as this, it is important to supplement your diet with iron and zinc as well as other vitamins and minerals that naturally accompany protein foods. (There is a fuller discussion of vitamin/mineral supplementation later in this chapter.)

Protein sources

The best low-fat protein sources are fat-free dairy products (milk, yogurt, and cottage cheese); "fake" meats made from soy; and pure protein pills (amino acid tablets). Other sources of protein, such as meats; peas, beans, and lentils; and tofu, are somewhat higher in protein but also higher in fat. Many whole grains contain a small amount of protein as well. If you eat meat, insist that it be as lean as possible.

Carbohydrates

These are the best source of calories to fuel your muscles and brain. If your body has to burn protein or fat for fuel, toxic by-products are formed. We do not recommend low-carbohydrate diets for this reason. Instead, we recommend getting about 55% of daily calories from carbohydrate foods such as vegetables, peas and beans, fruits, bread, pasta, and cereal. Whenever possible, use whole-grain products with reduced amounts of added saturated fats. These products are higher in B vitamins, other nutrients that are believed to help relieve arthritis symptoms.

Fiber

Here is another good reason to concentrate on carbohydrates: High-carbohydrate foods such as fruits, vegetables, and whole grains are also usually high in fiber. Recent research has suggested that changes in the intestinal bacteria population associated with a diet high in whole grains, fruits, and vegetables plays an important role in relieving rheumatoid arthritis symptoms. Also, a high-fiber diet contributes to long-term cardiovascular health by lowering insulin levels. A high intake of fiber in the diet is also associated with lower weight.

Fats

Animal fats such as butter, lard, and meat fat contain arachidonic acid, which is a key step in the metabolic chain resulting in the body's inflammation response. For this reason, many experts and patients agree that some people with rheumatoid arthritis can benefit from a vegan diet — one that is completely lacking in animal products. (See Chapter 9 for a fuller discussion.) Saturated fats are also well known to contribute to heart disease and some cancers. Also, commonly used vegetable oils such as corn, sunflower, and safflower are easily converted to the same arachidonic acid. Thus, a sensible dietary modification is to strictly limit saturated fats (including palm and coconut oil, which are often found in baked goods); change your vegetable oil to olive and canola (especially for high-temperature cooking); and make sure to add flaxseed oil (especially for low-temperature cooking and uncooked uses such as salad dressings). These modifications not only will help to reduce inflammation, pain, and stiffness, but also are good for your heart and arteries.

If you are on a weight loss regimen, it is very important to limit all fats. Vegetable fats such as grain, seed, and nut oils tend to be less saturated and less harmful than animal fats such as butter and margarine, but they are equally calorie-dense. Try to limit all fats to no more than 20% of total calories, which is equal to 240 calories on a 1200-calorie diet. This amounts to about 27 grams of total fat, or 2.5 tablespoons per day.

How to Create a Balanced Diet

If you are like most Americans, your diet is excessively high in fats, especially saturated fats from meat, baked goods, and butterfat, and also too high in protein. While the excess protein intake may not do any harm, the excess fat harms in many ways, causing inflammation through the arachidonic acid pathway, adding excess weight, and increasing the risk of heart disease, to name a few. Balancing your diet usually requires making some or all of the following changes:

• Eat a wide variety of foods.

• Match your food intake with your level of physical activity.

Vegetarianism

Throughout this chapter I will be emphasizing a healthy vegetarian diet. That is what I have followed for over 45 years, and it is traditionally how serious Yoga students eat, because it is a nonviolent diet. You do not have to be a vegetarian to practice Yoga, but this type of diet may actually help relieve arthritis symptoms (see Chapter 9). It is heartening to me that, after years of vegetarianism being regarded as somewhat "kooky," science has proven that a vegan, vegetarian, or mostly vegetarian diet often reduces arthritis symptoms. Many other chronic conditions are also reduced or even prevented by a diet rich in whole grains, and fruits and vegetables. It is also true that a healthy vegetarian diet helps you lose weight, because it gives you a greater volume of food to eat, since meat products are so calorie-dense.

• Choose a diet with plenty of grain products, vegetables, and fruits.

• Choose a diet low in total fat, and especially low in saturated fat and cholesterol.

• Eat only moderate amounts of sugar, salt, and processed foods with added sodium.

• Moderate your intake of alcohol.

If your diet has been severely imbalanced for a long time, it may take a while for your body to respond. Don't be discouraged; instead of thinking "I am dieting," think: "I am eating today the way I want to be eating next year and the year after." Go for the long term, not the short term.

I want to advise you to approach changes in your eating habits very slowly. Try to make one or two incremental steps each week. This will enable you to succeed in small ways every day. Gradually, you will easily be able to set your daily goal and happily stay with it. If you suddenly impose rigid requirements on yourself, both the inner and outer body are likely to rebel and sabotage your efforts.

Here is an easy way to get started: For the first week, replace three items that are high in saturated fats with low-fat replacements. Make it easy on yourself. For instance, if you want ice cream for dessert, eat frozen, fat-free yogurt instead. Replace a high-fat pastry with a low-fat whole-grain one. Snack on carrots or a piece of an apple instead of chips or salted nuts. Realize carefully what you have done and cajole both bodies with the inner conversation that you have given your physical body what it wants and that you are also proud and appreciative of the emotional support that was provided from the inner body.

The Yoga Arthritis Diet

We are basing our suggestions for the anti-arthritis diet on the USDA Food Guide Pyramid, which suggests how to build your daily diet in terms of servings of different food groups. Before setting out the specific diet plan, I want to tell you more about the Food Guide Pyramid and offer some general suggestions about reducing fat and sugar in your diet.

The Food Guide Pyramid

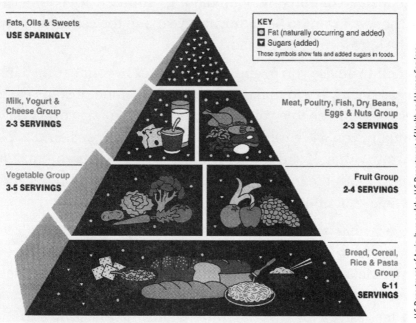

Fats, Oils & Sweets
USE SPARINGLY

KEY
▢ Fat (naturally occurring and added)
▼ Sugars (added)
These symbols show fats and added sugars in foods.

Milk, Yogurt & Cheese Group
2-3 SERVINGS

Meat, Poultry, Fish, Dry Beans, Eggs & Nuts Group
2-3 SERVINGS

Vegetable Group
3-5 SERVINGS

Fruit Group
2-4 SERVINGS

Bread, Cereal, Rice & Pasta Group
6-11 SERVINGS

U.S. Department of Agriculture and the U.S. Department of Health and Human Services

Starting from the lowest, widest level, the food guide pyramid emphasizes carbohydrates, allowing the greatest number of servings for these healthy fuel foods:

Grains:
Bread, cereal, rice, and pasta: 6 - 11 servings

Fruits and vegetables:
Vegetables: 3 - 5 servings
Fruits: 2 - 4 servings

Protein:
Dairy: 2 - 3 servings
Meat, poultry, fish,
dry beans, eggs, & nuts: 2 - 3 servings

Fats, oils, and sweets:
Small amounts of oil required to reduce inflammation. Use others sparingly.

How Many Servings Are Right for You?

If you are older, small in stature, inactive, a chronic dieter, athletic, female, or have a low metabolic rate, you probably have a really hard time maintaining ideal weight, possibly even gaining weight on a diet that helps your friends to lose weight! Doubtless, you should lean toward the low end of the range of servings per day.

On the other hand, bigger (by weight) and younger people, or those who are moderately to very active can afford to eat a higher number of daily servings. Also, men tend to have higher metabolic rates and can tolerate more servings than women.

What Is a Serving?

We have listed below some common foods and have separated out for your convenience some of the lower calorie options in each pyramid level. Because calorie counts for different foods vary widely, we suggest that you choose your foods mostly from the lower calorie groups if you, like most, need to shed excess pounds. Foods in the "other" category tend to be higher in calories and are more suitable if you are near your ideal weight and are careful to burn off excess calories with briskly paced exercise. Here are some examples from each group (see Resources for a list of books and Internet sites to use to find your own calorie counts):

Grains:

Low-calorie (avg. 70 cal./serv.)	Other (avg. 100 cal.)
Bow-tie pasta (1/2 c)	Elbow macaroni (1/2 c)
Weight Watchers oat bran bread (1 slice)	Raisin bread (1 slice)
Total Multigrain cornflakes (1 c)	Cheerios (1 c)
Cooked cereal (1/2 c)	White short- grain rice (1 c)

Vegetables (1/2 c servings unless otherwise noted):

Low calorie (avg. 17 cal.)	Other (avg. 64 cal.)
Asparagus	Winter squash
Broccoli	Corn
Beans, green	Peas

Cauliflower	Tomato sauce (canned)
Zucchini	Potato w/skin (1 med)

Fruits:

Low calorie (avg. 40 cal.)	**Other (avg. 102 cal.)**
Apple (1 med)	Apricots, dried (10 halves)
Blueberries (1/2 c)	Pear (1 med)
Grapes (10)	Banana (1 med)
Honeydew melon (1/8 melon)	Raisins (1/4 c)

Dairy:

Low calorie (avg. 90 cal.)	**Other (avg. 180 cal.)**
Skim milk (1 c)	Whole milk (1 c)
Plain yogurt (1 c)	Fruited nonfat yogurt (1 c)
2% cottage cheese (1/2 c)	Parmesan cheese (2 oz)
Light Swiss cheese (1 oz)	Cheddar cheese (1 oz)

Protein:

Low calorie (avg. 113 cal.)	**Other (avg. 189 cal.)**
Tofu, firm (3 oz)	Tempeh (4 oz)
Yves veg. weiner (1)	Chicken broiled (3 oz)
Yves Canadian bacon (4 slices)	Hamburger broiled (3 oz)
Dried beans (1/2 c cooked)	Beef, lean roasted (3 oz)

How to Reduce Inflammatory Fats

As I mentioned previously, many studies have shown that most animal fats (from meat and dairy foods) in your diet can increase your body's inflammatory reaction, making arthritis symptoms worse. Here are some suggestions on how to reduce these fats to help yourself lose excess pounds and help your heart at the same time.

Did you know that our taste preference for fatty foods is mostly learned? That means it can be unlearned. Many of my students and I have experienced this in our own lives as we have tried to improve our diets. For instance, many people used to dislike the taste of fat-free milk. By gradually switching to lower fat products, first 2%, then 1%, and finally fat-free, they found that eventually they preferred the taste of the fat-free product and did not miss the unnecessary additional butterfat. Recently some milk producers have improved skim milk simply by adding fat-free milk solids, resulting in even better taste and more fat-free protein and calcium, too; choose these brands whenever you can. Other culturally ingrained habits, such as butter on toast, full-fat ice cream, and sour cream on baked potatoes, can also be changed. My meat-eating friends tell me they have easily re-learned to prefer the taste of the leanest meats.

I think it is heartening to find out that when we take pains to break these saturated fat habits, we find that we prefer the taste and texture of foods without the added fat. Take a "fat vacation" for a month, and then see what fats you really cannot live without. Add the "must haves" back as sparingly as possible. If you are like most, you can enjoy food and the eating experience just as much with markedly less fat than you are used to. Here's how to reduce fats in the major food groups of the pyramid:

No-Fat Foolery

Remember that fat-free does not mean calorie-free! Many packaged items increase sugars and other calorie-dense ingredients in order to compensate for the reduced fat in their product. Read labels, and try to avoid eating packaged foods as much as possible. Especially enjoy the labels on such products as chocolate syrup and even apples, which say "as always, fat-free"!

First, let's talk about grains. How can we make sure this carbohydrate foundation to our diet is not too high in fat? First, try taking the "no-spread pledge." This means eating breads and toast without spreading on the butter or margarine. When eating breakfast in a restaurant, remember to ask for "dry whole wheat toast, please." If at first you can't face toast with no spread at all, try a small amount of no-added-sugar preserves or fat-free cream cheese. It is easy to find a cereal without added sugar, and simply by switching to fat-free milk, you are well on the way toward a really low-fat, low-calorie breakfast.

Do you always put gravy or butter on rice? Try serving rice as many Asians do, as a layer under low-fat vegetables or beans, peas, or lentils. Pasta dishes can be low-fat or high-fat items depending on the sauce. Do you know that Italian-style canned tomato pasta sauces vary from 0% to at least 50% of calories from fat? Many of the fat-free varieties are quite tasty and are widely available at major supermarkets. Remember, if it is a creamy pasta sauce, it probably is high-fat, and saturated to boot. If you really prefer the taste of a creamy sauce, sauté vegetables in a small amount of oil (use a canola oil spray) and stir fat-free yogurt into the pan after taking it off the heat, to make a low-fat creamy pasta topping. You can also try the more traditional approach of tossing the hot pasta and the sautéed vegetables with skim-milk ricotta cheese.

Unfortunately, there is no easy way to reduce the fat in cakes, cookies, and muffins unless you bake them yourself, although low-fat or fat-free products are increasingly available at local supermarket bakeries. If you do your own baking, you can substitute nonfat yogurt or applesauce for some or all of the butter or oil in the recipe. If high-fat foods such as pie crusts, croissants, and doughnuts are on your list of "must-haves," you'll have to limit them to once a week or less in order to truly benefit from a low-fat diet.

How about vegetables? Frying vegetables of any kind moves them from the highly recommended list all the way to the "use sparingly" list. The same for butter or cheese sauces for vegetables. Flavor your veggies with fresh herbs, lemon juice, and a little salt and pepper, or cook them with onions and garlic. Sauté them quickly in a nonstick pan, with perhaps a quick blast from a canola oil spray. Even the large portabello mushroom can be pan grilled this way. If a butter sauce is on your list of "must haves," try one of the instant natural butter flavor mixes.

Fruits are perhaps the best food for an arthritis diet because they are naturally full of carbohydrates, have a sweet taste, and are usually eaten with no added fat. The only fatty fruit habit that could be a problem is peanut butter on bananas.

At the dairy level of the pyramid, milk and yogurt are readily available in a range of fat content from 0% to 4%, and some brands of cottage, ricotta, and even Swiss, cheddar, and mozza-

How To Cheat!

First, don't call it cheating; call it being kind to both your bodies. If you find yourself really hungry, don't give up. Eat an extra grain serving along with a small serving of a protein-rich food; for example, a piece of good bread with a glass of fat-free milk. Avoid telling yourself "I've failed, I've blown it, there's no point in continuing," because you have not failed. You have begun a new relationship with your emotional body in a new awareness of its need to be happy. Second, avoid eating fatty foods; even in small portions they won't be as satisfying as a larger portion of carbohydrate and protein. Remember, carbohydrate foods are much less likely to be stored as body fat than the same calories from fatty foods.

rella cheeses are available in fat-free form. We were delighted to discover that even half-and-half has a new fat-free form, although it still contains over 50% more calories than fortified skim milk.

Now we come to a very difficult group — one that is often loaded with fat built right into the foods themselves. Meat, poultry, and fish dishes usually contain high amounts of saturated fat unless special efforts are made to purchase and prepare low-fat versions of typical recipes. Dried beans are traditionally cooked with added fat, egg yolks are high in cholesterol, which is a form of fat, and nuts are so high in fat they are even a good commercial source of oil. Perhaps peas and lentils are not so often loaded up with added fats as the other members of the group, but even here caution is needed. Split pea soup is traditionally prepared with added meat fat, and Indian methods of cooking the various legumes (dal) usually call for flavoring with clarified butter (ghee). In order to limit nonessential fat in this group, choose well-trimmed, low-fat meat, skinless poultry, grilled skinless fish, poached or boiled eggs (no more than three to four per week unless you use plain egg whites), nontraditional fat-free preparations of peas, beans, and lentils, and very limited amounts of nuts. Many of my friends who are trying to eat less meat complain, perhaps rightly so, about the inconvenience of soaking and simmering dried beans and lentils. There is often a slight shocked expression when I admit to using and enjoying the canned varieties.

Soy products are increasingly in evidence in major supermarkets, and their low-fat or nonfat varieties are an excellent source of protein. Certainly the "fake meat" wieners, burgers, Canadian bacon, and deli slices are healthier for you than the meats they mimic. Even if you are not a vegetarian, you will benefit from adding some of these foods to your diet; eating a "veggie" hot dog or slice of "veggie" bacon as a snack is a great comfort for hunger pangs. Most people are familiar with soybean curd (tofu), a staple food of Asia; it is a bland cakelike high-protein food that can be barbecued, scrambled, sautéed with vegetables, boiled, or baked. When processed with calcium, as it usually is, tofu is a great source of this essential mineral as well as protein. Although nearly 50% of tofu's calories are from fat, the fat is predominantly unsaturated.

Eating in Restaurants

Most restaurants, especially the fast-food establishments, seem to specialize in adding fat to foods in order to enhance the taste. Serving sizes have also grown and grown; in some major chains the amount of food on your plate can easily contain a whole day's requirements of calories. I remember well when a dietician, noting a major food chain's newest big burger, remarked that of course it wasn't too high in fat: just buy one on Monday, cut it into five pieces and eat a piece every day! Fried foods top the list of favorite restaurant foods. If it's fried, it's high in fat, and if it's batter-fried, it's doubly high. That also goes for refried items, cheese sauces, melted cheese, or cream sauce. Almost any whitish dipping sauce is code for mayonnaise, which means vegetable oil. Always ask for salad dressing on the side, and use as little as you can. You may discover you actually like and prefer the unadorned taste of vegetables.

When you order breakfast toast, forget about the yellow-colored fat carefully brushed from crust to crust; ask for dry toast and add your own butter or margarine or preserves, sparingly. Sometimes dry whole wheat toast and poached eggs are the only low-fat choices available. Granola is too often a blatant contradiction: widely associated with health, it is often high in both added fat and sugar. Pancakes can be a good choice, especially if you can find some with fiber, such as buckwheat, and limit the amount of added fat (butter, margarine) and sugar (syrup, jelly) you add.

Lunch can include salads, bread, and baked potatoes at most establishments. Deli sandwiches can be improved by replacing mayonnaise with mustard, adding more lettuce and tomato, using whole-grain bread products, and removing half the cheese or meat filling. Chinese food can be a good alternative if you select stir-fried vegetable and bean curd dishes with plain rice. Mexican food should probably be saved for rare special occasions; fried and refried foods are the order of the day; even avo-

Feeding Both Your Bodies

If you are faced with a high-fat burrito, taco, or other food, divide it into three parts. Eat one for your emotional body, one for your physical body, and then fantasize stuffing the other part into your unwilling hips and waist as they protest. If your emotional body fights for more, mark your wrist tape (see page 154) and figure out how to make up the loss to it. This will show you if you are constantly denying your inner emotional body and help you to notice when it rebels. This technique will work with any high-fat or high-sugar foods; you can even divide up all your meals this way just for fun.

cados are 93% calories from fat. Try to order plain flour tortillas, rice, and beans, and remove extra cheese from items such as tostados, tacos, burritos, and enchiladas. Go easy on the fried corn chip basket offered while you wait.

I do not recommend eating fewer than 1,200 calories per day without strict physician supervision, even though fasting has often been shown to reduce rheumatoid arthritis symptoms. Fasting and extremely low-calorie diets have severe effects on your body's metabolism; if you wish to lose excess weight, you may need to boost your activity level so that you can lose weight on 1,200 calories. Remember that strengthening, aerobic, and range-of-motion exercises are all required elements of arthritis self-help. These activities also increase your muscle mass and metabolic rate, which helps to keep weight off for the long term. For each 30 minutes of brisk activity each day, you can add back 135 calories (180 for men). Additional exercise is the best solution also for smaller people who hit the 1,200-calorie limit, because they can increase weight loss goals without reducing calories to dangerous levels.

Sample Menus

Following are two sample menus, the first for about 1,200 calories, and the second for 1,400 calories. You can easily adjust your calorie level upward by substituting an "other" choice for a low-calorie choice, or by adding 100 calories or so in a favorite snack. (See Resources for some excellent books and Internet sources that can help you create your own menus.)

Sample Menu for 1200 Calories

Breakfast

1c milk (fortified skim)	110	1 dairy
1c Product 19 cereal	100	1 grain
1/2 small banana	60	1 fruit
1/2 bagel	80	1 grain
	———	
	350	

Lunch

1/2 c tomato soup	90	1 veg
2 slices Weight Watcher's Oat bran bread	80	2 grain
4 slices Yves Veggie Pepperoni	90	1 protein

lettuce/tomato	25	1 veg
mustard	--	--
1/2 c melon	30	1 fruit
	———	
	315	

Snack

1 c yogurt — plain or artificially sweetened, nonfat	90	1 dairy

Dinner

Omelet made with 2 egg substitutes and 1/2 c veggies and 1 slice veg. Can. bacon	182	2 protein, 1 veg
1 tsp butter	45	1 fat
1 c mixed green salad	25	1 veg
2 Tbs fat free dressing	45	
1 slice whole-wheat toast	86	1 grain
1 tsp low-sugar spread	25	
	———	
	408	

Snack

2 rice cakes	80	1 grain
	———————	

1243 Total Calories

Sample Menu for 1400 Calories

Breakfast

Breakfast burrito	230	1 protein, 1 grain
Milk, 1 c	110	1 dairy
Papaya, 1/2 med	60	1 fruit
	——	
	400	

Lunch

Veggie Burger, Morningstar Farms	70	1 protein
Bun	60	2 grain
Kraft fat-free Swiss, 1 slice	30	1 dairy
Red onion, tomatoes	29	1 veg
Mixed green salad	19	1 veg
Fat-free dressing	33	
Peach	37	1 fruit
	——	
	278	

Snacks

Snack Wells fat free crackers (5)	60	1 grain
Carrot sticks and fat-free Vegetable dip	109	1 veg
	——	
	169	

Dinner

Ziti (1 c) with zucchini 1/2 c	232	2 grain, 1 veg
1 TB Parmesan ch	100	
Fruit salad, 1 c	101	2 fruit
Whole wheat roll	74	1 grain
1 c V-8 Juice	56	1 veg
	–––	
	563	

1410 Total Calories

Supplementing Your Diet for Arthritis

Food First!

Vitamin and mineral supplements cannot replace food. Foods have hundreds of yet-to-be-discovered chemicals that may be important to health; vitamin and mineral supplements have only a handful. It is best to eat a wide variety of foods and to avoid chemical excesses and imbalances. Don't be one of the 9 out of 10 Americans who do not regularly eat the recommended number of daily servings of fruits and vegetables, because research has clearly linked a high intake of these foods rich in vitamins C, E, beta-carotene, and other antioxidants with a markedly reduced risk of osteoarthritis. The best strategy for optimal health and reducing your risk of chronic diseases such as arthritis is to obtain adequate nutrients from a wide variety of foods.

Having said that, there are some instances in which supplementation may be a wise course. If you are severely restricting calories to lose weight, vitamins and minerals may well be undersupplied. Even a well-balanced diet can be lacking in adequate amounts if you restrict quantity and portion size. Generally, if you tend to skip meals, diet often, or eat meals high in sugar and fat, supplements are a reasonable course.

Who Should Supplement?

Many experts believe that chronic health problems — arthritis being perhaps preeminent — are related to a long-term nutritional imbalance: the body is unable to repair tissue as fast as it is damaged by wear and tear. For arthritis, it is imperative to focus on all aspects of diet affecting the body's ability to rebuild damaged joint tissue and to reduce inflammation. Safe and effective nutritional supplements are an important part of this strategy.

As I mentioned previously, the older population most at risk for arthritis is also most likely to be overweight and restricting food intake to lose weight. Older people often have irregular eating habits and do not eat a well-balanced diet, even when not restricting calories. Depression, lack of appetite, loss of taste and smell, and denture problems can all contribute to an older person not eating well. Absorption of vitamins can be impaired in older people. Older women often need extra vitamin D and calcium for protection from osteoporosis.

Women have special needs throughout life, starting with calcium and vitamin D to prevent osteoporosis. As I mentioned previously, lower levels of these nutrients increase arthritis risk, and arthritis affects twice as many older women as men. Women of child-bearing years usually do not get enough folic acid, which reduces neurological birth defects. Doctors usually prescribe vitamin and mineral supplements for pregnant and lactating women, whose requirements are higher during this time.

Vegans (vegetarians who eat absolutely no animal products, including dairy and eggs) are unlikely to get adequate amounts of vitamins D, B-2, and B-12, or calcium, iron, and zinc, and should consider supplementation. Please see the following chapter, starting on page 206, for helpful information about how to make a vegan diet nutritionally sound, because a vegan diet may help as many as 4 of 10 rheumatoid arthritics with symptomatic relief.

Best Food Sources — Vitamins

Here is a simple rule of thumb for getting your vitamin requirements from food: grains for B-complex, fruits and vegetables for vitamins A, C, and E. Citrus, bananas, cantaloupe, and dried fruits are all excellent; the vegetables with the highest vitamin content are always the most colorful ones. Dark green leafy vegetables such as spinach, colorful peppers, and all the members of the cabbage family such as broccoli, cauliflower, Brussels sprouts, and cabbage itself, along with carrots and winter squash, are all excellent sources.

All B-complex vitamins are included in whole-grain products except for B-12, which is found in milk, eggs, and meat. Eggs also supply most of the other B-complex vitamins, as do many fruits, vegetables, and meat. Vitamin D is added to milk and is formed on the skin by sunlight. Everyone should take a supplement with 400 mcg of folic acid, and most multivitamins include it.

Best Food Sources — Minerals

Iron is found in high amounts in beef and pork and in moderate amounts in prunes, apricots, spinach, beans, tofu, blackstrap molasses, nutritional yeast, and wheat germ. However, all sources are dwarfed by the iron content of fortified cereals. For example, a serving of Total brand cereal contains 18 mg of iron, which is 100% of the recommended daily intake. Younger people, especially premenopausal women, need the full amount of iron, but older men and women should be okay with 10 mg or less daily.

Zinc is much more difficult to obtain, with only beef, pork, and shellfish being good sources. Wheat germ, garbanzo beans, and lentils are the best of the rest, but in order to get the recommended 15 mg, you would need to eat nearly 1 1/2 cups of wheat germ, for instance. A mineral supplement supplying the recommended amount of zinc seems to make good sense, and again, most multivitamin/mineral supplements include the recommended amount.

Calcium is highest in dairy foods — milk, yogurt, and cheese — and other good sources include tofu (if processed with calcium sulfate) and dark green leafy vegetables (spinach, turnip greens, kale, etc.). Unless you commit to eating at least four servings per day of high-calcium dairy foods (1 serving = 1 cup milk, 1 cup yogurt, 1 oz hard cheese), a calcium supplement should be used to replace each missing high-calcium serving. Calcium supplements should usually total 900 - 1,000 mg (three 300 mg tablets or two 500 mg tablets daily) for older people.

Magnesium is an important part of calcium metabolism, affects nerves, and also reduces the risk of diabetes. Many studies indicate that Americans get too little. Whole grains and beans are the best sources, especially if they were grown in magnesium-rich soils. I take a calcium supplement that includes magnesium (about 1:3 or 1:2 magnesium-to-calcium ratio) for convenience, as the amount of magnesium in most multivitamin/mineral supplements is inadequate and the magnesium content of the soil my food is grown in is unknown.

Trace minerals are difficult to evaluate and should be sufficient in the diet provided unrefined foods such as whole grains and fresh fruits and vegetables provide the majority of calories. The single exception is selenium. Add 200 mcg selenium to your supplement list for protection from prostate, lung, and colon cancers; again, most multivitamin/mineral supplements contain this amount.

Dietary Supplements and Arthritis

The basic diet includes recommendations for good mulitvitamin/mineral supplements. This should be boosted with higher levels of several vitamins and minerals to help protect joints and perhaps even allow for some repair and rebuilding of eroded cartilage. Most important, studies often show that arthritic joint fluid is low in antioxidants, which means that cartilage repair processes are impaired. The vitamins A, E, and C and the mineral selenium are the principal antioxidants, so it's smart to increase them to higher levels. For vitamin A it's best to depend on a diet rich in beta-carotene-containing fruits and vegetables such as cantaloupe, carrots, and sweet potatoes, and limit supplements to a total daily amount of 15,000 IU (for osteoarthritis).

There are a host of other natural antioxidants in the news (lutein, beta-cryptoxanthine, flavinoids, lycopene, etc). All of them — and countless others as yet undiscovered by marketers — are available in plant foods, especially darkly colored fruits and vegetables. You must make sure that you include at least five servings of these in your diet every day, and our basic diet includes these. All good-quality multivitamin/mineral supplements contain 5,000 IU of vitamin A, so add 10,000 IU of beta-carotene daily to achieve the 15,000 suggested amount. Vitamin C needs to be supplied up to 500 to 1,000 mg daily in order to saturate all the tissues. More than this is simply excreted. The best plan is to take 500 mg twice daily. Multivitamins usually contain only a small fraction of this amount. Vitamin E benefits seem to increase with daily amounts in capsule form up to 400 to 600 IU, and again, more isn't more. Multivitamins usually contain 30 to 60 IU. Calcium, magnesium, and vitamin D are all critical for bone health and often need to be supplemented: 1,000 to 1,200 mg daily, 300 mg per dose, from citrate for calcium and 1/3 to 1/2 that for magnesium. Vitamin D is included in most multivitamins and added to many dairy products.

See page 187 for a suggested daily supplement schedule.

Supplement Quality and Dosages

I usually go to large retailers where the price is lowest: Wal-Mart or Kmart, for example. The vitamin and mineral compounds in all supplements are manufactured by a small group of multinational corporations such as ADM, and "natural" vitamins are no better in quality. Many supplements include additives such as herbs and enzymes, but they contain these elements in such tiny amounts that they can do you no real good.

The only quality issues for supplements are (1) nutrient content (does the tablet contain the labeled amount?), (2) whether the tablet will dissolve properly, and (3) purity. Although there are no federal standards for vitamins, you can help ensure quality by looking for the letters "USP" on the bottle, which indicates voluntary compliance with U. S. Pharmacopoeia, and by sticking to major brands; "store" brands are usually good bargains.

I usually take vitamin/mineral supplements after a meal for better absorption, and I take E and calcium at a different time of day than the basic multivitamin that includes iron. This is because calcium interferes with iron absorption, and iron may rapidly oxidize the vitamin E. Some experts suggest not taking vitamins and minerals at the same time as any prescription medications, so wait a few hours between to reduce the risk of interference. The basic multivitamin/minerals can cost as little as 10 cents or less per day, or as much as 50 cents or even higher for designer brands, though, as I mentioned earlier, there is no noticeable advantage to buying the higher priced brands.

Here are three steps to ensure you are getting an adequate amount of essential vitamins, minerals, and other vital cartilage-building nutrients:

1. The best choice is to eat moderate amounts of a wide variety of foods prepared in such a way as to preserve the naturally occurring vitamins and minerals. The most nutritious foods are fat-free dairy products; deeply colored fruits and vegetables such as carrots, spinach, apricots, mangos, winter squash, and tomatoes; whole-grain bread and cereal products; and good protein sources such as soy-based meat substitutes, dried beans and peas, and, if you eat meat, the leanest possible cuts of meat, poultry, and fish. If some of the choices mentioned here don't sound appetizing to you, do some research and find some nu-

tritious alternatives that you do like. It's important to eat food that you enjoy. This type of diet supplies a vast range of naturally occurring vitamins, minerals, and other compounds that science is just now learning about, such as flavinoids and phytoestrogens, that can never be included in a supplement tablet. Fruits and vegetables should be eaten raw, steamed, or quickly sautéed to preserve nutrients, as frying, boiling, and baking tend to destroy nutrient value. The nutrients in meat products are pretty much immune to such destruction, and grains usually must be boiled or baked for digestibility.

2. After you have fully established your new, more wholesome diet, consider taking a complete multivitamin/mineral supplement daily. Look for those that provide at least 100% of the daily value for A, B-1, B-2, niacin, B-6, B-12, C, D, E, and folic acid. Limit beta carotene to no more than 15,000 IU, iron to 18 mg, phosphorous to 500 mg, and B-6 to 200 mg. The supplement should also provide at least 25 mcg of vitamin K, 120 mcg of chromium, 100 mg magnesium, 2 mg copper, and 15 mg zinc. Iron requirements vary with gender and age. Women under 50 need 8 to 18 mg of iron, men under 50 need under 10 mg, and men and women over 50 need no more than 10 mg iron. Everyone over 50 needs at least 24 mcg of B-12, because of generally poor absorption in older bodies. Everyone with arthritis should have plenty of the antioxidant selenium, so make sure there is at least 200 mcg included.

A comprehensive multivitamin/mineral is a simple and relatively inexpensive choice. As I discussed earlier, you do not need to spend a lot of money on a supplement; the cheapest "store" brands are often as well-balanced and effective as the more expensive brands. When I was eliminating artificial colors from my diet to relieve symptoms of rheumatoid arthritis, I learned to buy uncolored brands, or I rinsed the outer colored coating off, leaving the hard white shell on the tablets, before swallowing. Following are some recommended brands (valid at publication):

For Women — Centrum, Dr. Art Ulene Nutrition Boost Formula for Men & Women, Kroger Complete Extra, OneSource, Rite Aid Whole Source, Safeway Select Omnisource, Spring Valley Advantage, Summit Complete, Twinlab Dualtabs, Walgreens Ultra Choice, YourLife Super Multi-Vitamin.

For Men — Dr. Art Ulene Nutrition Boost Formula for Men & Women, Eckerd Daily Impact Senior, Rite Aid Whole Source Mature Adult, Safeway Select Omnisource Senior, Shaklee Vita-Lea without iron, Twinlab Dualtabs, YourLife Super Multi-vitamin.

For Older Men and Women (Over 50) — Dr. Art Ulene Nutrition Boost Formula for Men & Women, Eckerd Daily Impact Senior, Rite Aid Whole Source Mature Adult, Safeway Select Omnisource Senior, Twinlab Dualtabs. (Brand recommendations adapted from the newsletter *Nutrition Action* [see Resources], April 2000 issue.) At the time of publication, all of these selections cost less than $5 for a month's supply, except for the Shaklee and Twinlab products.

3. Boost the potency of the multivitamin/mineral supplement you have chosen. As mentioned previously, it is often useful to add more calcium, magnesium, vitamin C, and vitamin E to the daily multi described above. These nutrients are usually undersupplied in a multivitamin/mineral supplement, and they are vital for cartilage repair and protection. With the above exceptions in mind, it is a good idea to limit your intake of vitamins and minerals to no more than 150% of the RDA, as large

amounts of some vitamins and minerals can be toxic. The following table suggests how to take supplements throughout the day for best absorption (see Chapter 9 for more about glucosamine, chondroitin, and other supplements not discussed in this chapter):

Arthritis Supplements

Breakfast

> *Multivitamin/ mineral;*
> *300 mg calcium*
> *150 mg magnesium*
> *500 mg vitamin C*
> *500 mg glucosamine**
> *400 mg chondroitin*
> *Oil, MSM, or SAM on trial basis*

Lunch

> *300 mg calcium*
> *150 mg magnesium*
> *500 mg glucosamine*
> *400 mg chondroitin*
> *Same as above*

Supper

> *300 mg calcium*
> *150 mg magnesium*
> *1,000 mg vitamin C*
> *400 IU vitamin E*

500 mg glucosamine

400 mg chondroitin

Same as above

*Add 500 mg extra if over 200 pounds.

Chapter 9

Alternative Diets and Supplements for Arthritis

Medical attitudes concerning the ability of diet and dietary supplements to ameliorate arthritis symptoms began with "Absolutely not!," proceeded to "Well, possibly," and now have arrived at the current view: "Actually, there is quite a bit you can do!"

Especially in Europe, new kinds of dietary supplements, specifically glucosamine and/or chondroitin, have clearly demonstrated benefit. If you have arthritis, I recommend that you try glucosamine and chondroitin for at least three months to find out if these supplements will benefit you. Quite a bit of research has demonstrated the safety and effectiveness of these supplements. The only thing lacking now in the research is a realistic measure of how much benefit there actually is and who is likely to benefit most from the supplements.

In addition, you can add to your basic diet a number of safe nutritional alternatives that have helped many people, although there is no clear evidence yet that they are truly effective. These include high vitamin B-complex, high omega-3 oils, MSM, and SAM-e.

Finally, although difficult to document, people continue to report that they suffer from rheumatoid arthritis symptoms due to food allergies, as I did (see p. 204). The most common allergens are animal products such as meat and dairy products. One leading expert convincingly demonstrated this effect in 3 of 16 patients who claimed food sensitivity, and another careful test demonstrated significant benefit in 12 out of 27 rheumatoid arthritis patients following a strict vegan, gluten-free diet. In this second group, most of the benefits remained after participants changed to a more liberal vegetarian diet (including dairy products). In this chapter you will find guidelines for a vegan diet that is safe and nutritionally sound.

If you decide to try some of these alternate supplements or diets, the best way to begin is to try just one at a time, so you will have a better idea if it actually helps you. Any of these alternatives should be tried for about three months — ample time to detect benefit — and then discarded if not effective for you. Because arthritis is usually a chronic disease, it is likely that you will have plenty of time to check out various remedies and alternatives. Of course, never ever discard prescribed medications or treatments in favor of an alternative remedy that might be ineffective, as you may well experience irreversible joint damage without your prescribed medications.

Watch Out for Fad Diets

As yet there is no cure for arthritis, and if one comes along, you will have to be living on Mars to avoid hearing about it! When you read or hear about the latest "cure," give it careful consideration before rushing out to buy something that may help, but may also hurt. Here are some points to keep in mind when evaluating news of the latest arthritis cure:

1. Does it sound like a sales pitch, based on stories of miraculous cures? For decades, arthritis sufferers have been the target of fad diets and bogus cures. The fact that thousands of people have tried a new remedy and claim that it is safe does NOT prove it is safe! MSM is a good example: Thousands have used it, many claim that it has benefited them, but to date there has been no systematic medical follow-up in a clinical trial to look for either a benefit or possible hidden side effects. Thus it appears to be safe, but actually may not be. (See p. 00 for more about MSM.) A great sage once said words to the effect that you can find 50 examples of anything, so don't be misled by anecdotes and testimony.

2. Other important questions to ask are: Is it a one-food or miracle-food diet? Does it promise a cure? Does the diet provide adequate nutrition? Highly restrictive diets cannot possibly meet nutritional requirements, nor are you likely to be able to stand it for more than a few days. Nutritional adequacy is imperative and is based on a number of factors, principally including a wide variety of foods rich in vitamins and minerals. Be wary of fad diets based on single substances that have not been proven to be at least safe, if not effective.

If you opt to try an alternative remedy, don't keep it a secret from your physician, as there are occasional drug interactions that should be considered.

Glucosamine and Chondroitin

The goal in dietary help for arthritis is to provide your body with all the nutrients necessary to "rev up" cartilage repair and protect joint tissues from being torn down. Two compounds, glucosamine and chondroitin, have been proven to not only safely benefit osteoarthritis symptoms, but also to show promise of actually improving joint health. Both glucosamine and chondroitin resemble molecules present in cartilage, and may provide the building blocks needed for repair and rebuilding. Cartilage tissue (like most other parts of the body) is constantly being torn down and replaced; in osteoarthritis, the repair process is simply outstripped by the tearing down process.

Chondroitin sulfate is a compound found throughout your body, occurring naturally in cartilage, where it seems to draw in and hold fluid to keep joints flexible and well lubricated. Supplements have been used in Europe for years, and are made from bovine cartilage. It appears to help reduce joint deterioration, increase flexibility and strength, and also ease pain. Chondroitin is slow acting; it takes at least two months for effects to show, so give it a try for at least three months before deciding if it helps you. Most people take three doses during the day of 400 mg each.

Glucosamine helps the pain and stiffness of osteoarthritis, containing the building blocks for making and repairing cartilage, and it has been used for more than a decade in Europe to treat osteoarthritis. Supplements are currently made from the shells of common shellfish. In the joints, it is a component of proteoglycan, which the body uses to build and repair cartilage. It helps ease the pain of osteoarthritis as well as the NSAIDs (especially ibuprofen) do, and has significantly fewer side effects.

It will be years before studies are concluded to tell if the substance actually helps rebuild damaged cartilage. Results so far indicate that it is most useful for those with mild to moderate cartilage loss. Take three doses daily of 500 mg each (four 500 mg each per day if you weigh over 200 pounds). Glucosamine is available in both sulfate and hydrochloride forms, and they appear to work equally well.

Although they are not considered essential nutrients in the same sense as vitamins and minerals from healthy food, both chondroitin and glucosamine sulfates have convincingly demonstrated both efficacy and safety in helping reduce arthritis symptoms. The March 15, 2000, issue of the *Journal of the American Medical Association* reported that both chondroitin and glucosamine are effective in treating osteoarthritis. After careful review of 13 clinical placebo-controlled, double-blind studies, scientists have concluded that these compounds are beneficial for osteoarthritis of the knee and hip. Glucosamine moderately reduced pain and improved function, while chondroitin had a large effect.

Researchers caution that the extent of the benefit of these compounds is as yet unknown, and they predict that it will be more modest than is claimed by some. The main problem is that most of these studies were supported by the manufacturers of the compounds, which usually means that if negative results are found, they tend to be minimized.

It is important to note that these products are not regulated by the FDA, so there is little guarantee that supplements actually contain the ingredients listed on the label. It is smart to choose products made by well-established manufacturers, and to buy them from reputable retailers. The two compounds are often combined in supplements, as well as sold individually, and there is no known synergy between the two. These compounds are widely available from pharmacies, health food stores, and large national retailers such as Wal-Mart and Kmart.

Although I recommend that anyone with arthritis add these compounds to the daily diet, it is still too early to actually insist on it. It's important to remember that not everyone with osteoarthritis will benefit from these compounds, because they are not "essential" in the same way that vitamins and minerals are. Also, we don't really know yet just how much benefit there is for different kinds or degrees of arthritis. To date, the only known side effects in people are occasional nausea or indigestion, which disappear either on their own or when the supplements are stopped.

There is no direct proof that the supplements rebuild or even slow cartilage loss in humans, but there is some evidence of these from both animal and lab studies, which gives support to the idea that human cartilage can be rebuilt.

High Vitamin B Complex

Several of the B vitamins help arthritis: Niacin (niacinamide or B-3) helps NSAIDs relieve pain and seems to improve joint mobility. Doses higher than about 500 mg daily may cause liver damage, but as little as 25 mg daily provided benefit in studies. Most multivitamins contain 20 mg, which is the recommended daily value. Some research has shown that pantothenic acid (B-5) has been some help, especially for rheumatoid arthritis. The daily value is only 10 mg, the amount found in a multivitamin, but levels up to even 2,000 mg appear to be safe, and the usual dose for people with rheumatoid arthritis is 250 mg daily. I have taken this amount twice daily when inflammation flares. Pyridoxine (B-6) and folic acid combine well together to reduce the risk of heart disease, which is sometimes associated with other forms of arthritis, and folic acid itself plays a key role in producing SAM (also called SAM-e; see p. 202), a cartilage-building joint compound. Also, people with rheumatoid arthritis who take methotrexate need extra folic acid because this drug reduces folic acid levels. More than 200 mg daily of B-6 may cause temporary nerve problems. People usually take about 50 mg of B-6 and 1 mg of folic acid daily, and schedule the folic acid around the methotrexate doses, according to their physician's direction.

Here are two possible ways to include extra B-complex vitamins in your daily intake:

Plan #1 — Maximum B-Complex

Take a high-potency B complex supplement: for example, a generic store brand with 50 mg of B-1, B-3, and B-5, 12 mg B-2 and B-6, 50 mcg folic acid, 12 mcg B-12, and 25 mcg biotin. Add a 400-mcg folic acid tablet and a 250-mg pantothenic acid capsule twice daily. Thus, your total B-complex intake for the day, combining your basic multivitamin, the high-potency B-complex supplement, and the extra pantothenic and folic acid supplements, gives you all the right amounts of the B-complex vitamins that may help arthritis, both osteo- and rheumatoid, in safe amounts. At worst, you have wasted some very small change; these higher doses are known to be harmless, and the tablets are not very expensive.

Plan #2 — Simple B-Complex

This plan provides the minimum amounts of only those B-complex vitamins known to have an impact on arthritis, with nothing else added. Simply add the following tablets/capsules to your basic multivitamin:10 mg niacinamide (B-3), 50 mg pyridoxine (B-6), 400 mcg folic acid, and one 250 mg pantothenic acid (B-5) capsule twice daily.

Neither plan, of course, replaces the basic multivitamin/mineral supplementation described in Chapter 8.

Essential Fatty Acids

Over the past decade, several promising animal and human studies have revealed that essential fatty acid (EFA) supplements help ease the symptoms of rheumatoid arthritis. Administration of various EFAs has resulted in improvement in joint strength and a decrease in joint pain, swelling, and morning stiffness in people with rheumatoid arthritis. More studies are needed to examine further the function, benefits, and dosages of EFAs in alleviating symptoms. But because there are few adverse effects from taking essential fatty acid supplements, many physicians support their use when combined with other arthritis therapies.

Several essential fatty acids contribute to the body's antiinflammation and immune system-regulating processes. This is achieved through complex chemical reactions that either inhibit or support the production of prostaglandins and other factors that increase or reduce inflammation. EFAs that help to reduce inflammation include gamma linolenic acid (GLA), eicosapentaenoic acid (EPA), docosahexaenoic acid (DHA), and alpha linolenic acid (ALA).

Several sources recommend diet supplementation with a combination of the above EFAs. Although not easily found in foods, GLA is found in large quantities in several plant seed oils, such as evening primrose, borage, and blackcurrant. EPA and DHA are prevalent in cold-water fish oils. There are no vegetarian food sources of EPA/DHA, with the exception of red and brown algae. However, ALA is metabolized by the body into EPA. Although this conversion is not 100% efficient, individuals who do not wish to take a fish oil supplement or who do not eat fish can substitute a plant seed oil that contains ALA, such as flaxseed. ALA is also found in dark green leafy vegetables, pumpkin seeds, walnuts, and several beans, including soy, kidney, lima, navy, and great northern. A word of caution regarding ALA supplementation: Digestion of common vegetable oils (corn, safflower, sunflower, etc.) uses the same enzymes that are needed to convert ALA to EPA. So, you also need to decrease your consumption of these vegetable oils by substituting olive or canola oil.

Flaxseed comes in various forms, as a liquid oil, as whole seeds, or in a flour. The oil can be used to make salad dressing and for sautéing, but not for high-temperature cooking. The seeds can be sprinkled on salads, cereals, or casseroles. The flour can be used in baking, by substituting some of the regular flour in a recipe with flaxseed flour. The recommended dosage of flaxseed is one to three tablespoons of oil per day, or about 30 grams (1/4 cup) of flour. If you need to lose excess pounds, limit yourself to just one tablespoon daily, as all oils contain about 100 calories per tablespoon.

Evening primrose or borage seed oil (borage seed oil has a higher concentration of GLA) can be taken in capsule form. A dosage of 1,800 mg of GLA per day is recommended. The number of capsules needed per day will depend upon the amount of active GLA in each capsule. Read the label carefully and calculate your intake accordingly; this small amount adds only a trivial amount of fatty calories to your diet.

As with all dietary supplements, it is best to begin with a low dosage and increase the dosage slowly until you see some benefit. Gastrointestinal upset and loose stools have been reported by some people who take EFA supplements. Increasing the dosage slowly will help your body adjust to the supplement and decrease the possibility of these side effects. One study reported that people did not see benefits until they had taken an EFA supplement for at least 6 to 12 weeks. In this study, benefits continued to increase the longer people took the supplement (18 to 24 weeks). If no benefit is noted after about three months, it is time to reassess whether EFA supplementation works for you.

Oils or capsules should be refrigerated and should be packaged in an opaque plastic container. Pay close attention to the expiration date on liquid oils and capsules. In order to ensure quality, I recommend that you try to buy plant oils that are certified organic and are "expeller-pressed," which means that no chemicals or heat were used in the manufacturing process.

It has been noted that fish oil and the GLA oils can act as blood thinners. This could increase the risk of bleeding for people who are also taking NSAIDs, aspirin, other blood-thinning medications that slow clotting. Although there were no reported incidents of bleeding in any of the studies on EFAs, be cautious. As with any new regimen, check with your doctor.

Balancing Dietary Fat Intake

In addition to supplementing your diet with the above EFAs, it is important to monitor all fat intake in your diet. It is well known that most Americans' diets contain too much fat. Much of this fat is of the omega-6 variety (most vegetable oils and animal fats such as butter and lard) that, when metabolized in the body, contributes to inflammation (with the exception of GLA). The omega-3 variety of fatty acids (ALA, DPA, and EPA sources as described above) do not have this effect. Although our bodies need both omega-3 and omega-6 oils (in a ratio of about 2:1), adjusting your diet to increase your intake of omega-3 and decrease your intake of omega-6 fatty acids may help in alleviating arthritis symptoms. Cooking with olive or canola oil, rather than corn or other vegetable oils, will increase your intake of omega-3s. Avoiding processed and fast foods will go a long way in helping to decrease your intake of omega-6 oils, as will the elimination of animal foods containing saturated fats (meat and butterfat). This is good advice not only for arthritis sufferers but also for anyone who is committed to maintaining good health and preventing the onset or progression of many diseases.

The new "fake fats," such as Olestra, bind with fat-soluble vitamins, antioxidants, and other important nutrients in the digestive tract. These are then passed out of the digestive system without being absorbed into and used by the body. This is clearly a detrimental effect, especially for those with certain disease conditions. As tempting as they may seem, foods containing these "fake fats" are not healthy and should not be a part of your diet or fat-reduction regimen.

Sulfur Compounds

Sulfur represents about 0.25% of total body weight. It is distributed in small amounts in all body cells and tissues, and is an important component of protein. It is present in four amino acids, including the essential amino acid methionine, and two B vitamins, thiamine and biotin. Sulfur plays a role in many physiologic functions relating to enzyme reactions, hormone balance, and protein synthesis.

Sulfur is important to the formation of the protein collagen, found in connective tissue. Sulfur is present in large quantities in joint tissues, in the form of chondroitin sulfate. Although it may be coincidental, it has been determined that the sulfur content of the fingernails of people with arthritis is often lower than normal. The following sulfur compounds may help to alleviate arthritis pain and joint inflammation.

MSM

MSM (methyl sulfonyl methane) is a sulfur compound found in many fresh fruits and vegetables, milk, eggs, grains, fish, and legumes. However, it is quickly destroyed by food processing, preparation, and storage. This may explain why diet alone does not provide sufficient quantities of MSM for some people. MSM has received considerable attention through numerous anecdotal reports of arthritis pain relief. There have been some animal studies of MSM that have shown relief of rheumatoid arthritis-type symptoms. At this time there are no published human studies regarding the safety, function, efficacy, or dosing of MSM. The main researcher on MSM, Stanley Jacobs, is the medical director of a company that sells MSM, so some critics believe that he is not totally objective.

The manufacturers of MSM currently market it for relief of both rheumatoid arthritis and osteoarthritis pain, and anecdotal reports are positive in MSM providing pain relief for both conditions. A great deal of publicity has recently been generated, mainly through a major testimonial from the actor James Coburn, who has rheumatoid arthritis, in an appearance on the Larry King Show. See Resources for web sites containing information from manufacturers, Mr. Coburn's testimonial, and a summary from the Arthritis Foundation. After checking out this information, I suggest making up your own mind on whether to give MSM a try or not, remembering that safety should be your highest priority. As of this writing, indications are that MSM will do no harm, and might do some people some good.

MSM is a normal oxidation product of DMSO (dimethyl sulfoxide). DMSO is a compound that has been studied in both animal and human subjects, and has been shown to relieve muscle and joint pain and inflammation. DMSO has been used for arthritis treatment for many years in other countries. It cannot be sold for this purpose in the United States, where it is approved by the FDA only for the treatment of interstitial cystitis (not as an oral preparation). MSM is reported by users to have many of the same beneficial effects as DMSO, but without side effects such as a bad taste in the mouth and a garlic-like skin odor. The researchers who discovered MSM believe the results of DMSO studies can be applied to MSM as well, because MSM is a natural derivative of DMSO. However, this view is not widely shared by rheumatologists and others in the field, who believe that human clinical studies must be conducted on MSM before it is proven to be beneficial and safe for arthritis treatment.

MSM is available in the United States as an over-the-counter dietary supplement. As it is touted as a good remedy for both pain and inflammation, it may be of benefit for both osteoarthritis and rheumatoid arthritis. If you wish to try MSM, I recommend that you begin with a low dosage (500 mg twice a day) and gradually increase the dosage until you note some effect. Most suppliers of MSM recommend a dosage of one to two grams (1,000-2,000 mg) two or three times a day. There may be some initial side effects, such as gastrointestinal upset, which should be reported to your physician if they persist. The beneficial effects of MSM may not appear for the first four to eight weeks. If you experience no pain relief after this initial period, MSM may not be beneficial for you specifically.

SAM-e

S-adenosyl-methionine (SAM, marketed as SAM-e) is another supplement that has been reported to help relieve arthritis pain and inflammation. SAM is a compound that occurs naturally in all human cells, a combination of the sulfur-containing amino acid methionine and adenosine triphosphate, ATP, the principal source of cellular energy. Among numerous physiologic functions, SAM plays an important role in the maintenance of cartilage in the joints.

Although our bodies generally manufacture SAM in sufficient amounts, some studies have shown that levels of SAM decrease with age. SAM levels may also be low in those with insufficient levels of B vitamins, especially folic acid, or the essential amino acid methionine.

SAM has been approved for use in 14 European countries for over 20 years, as a prescription medication for both arthritis and depression. It has been studied extensively in Europe in numerous controlled clinical trials. In 12 studies involving about 22,000 subjects, SAM was shown to be as effective as nonsteroidal anti-inflammatory drugs (NSAIDs) in relieving osteoarthritic pain, without the gastrointestinal side effects of NSAIDs. Although SAM has been shown to be safe over short-term therapy, there are currently no clinical trials studying the long-term effects of SAM use. There is no scientific evidence at this time to support the idea that SAM helps rebuild cartilage, although this is a claim of some manufacturers. Some researchers believe further studies may show that SAM does play a role in improving joint disease and rebuilding cartilage, as well as providing pain relief.

Studies indicate that 400 mg per day of SAM is an effective dosage for arthritis pain relief for most people (dosages as high as 1,600 mg per day were used in studies on the use of SAM for depression). As with all supplements, it is best to begin with a low dosage and increase the dose as needed until you see benefit, not exceeding the manufacturer's recommended maximum dosage. Use a full-strength SAM supplement, in the form of either tosylate or butanedisulfonate, from a reliable manufacturer. SAM supplements (usually called SAM-e) are widely available from pharmacies, major retailers, and health food stores in 200-mg tablets. Currently, SAM, at about $60 for one month's supply, is rather expensive.

Food Sensitivity and Rheumatoid Arthritis

Perhaps the principal controversy about diet and arthritis is the vast store of anecdotes relating how food sensitivities cause rheumatoid arthritis. Fingers have been pointed for decades at the nightshade family (potatoes, tomatoes, eggplant), animal products (both meat and dairy), and corn and wheat. Some well-known diets call for the elimination of all animal products from the diet, and also reduced fat.

Norman Childers was a horticulturist who suffered from severe rheumatoid arthritis. He noticed that his arthritis flared up whenever he ate tomatoes, so he decided to eliminate nightshades from his diet and noticed considerable improvement. Though Childers claimed to have worked with over 5,000 osteoarthritis and rheumatoid arthritis patients who benefited by eliminating nightshades, no credible research has since demonstrated a relationship between particular foods, especially the nightshades, and rheumatoid arthritis. Childers' theory was that chemical alkaloids contained in nightshades are deposited in the connective tissue, stimulating inflammation and inhibiting cartilage formation. Childers wrote about his findings in a book (now out of print) called *A Diet to Stop Arthritis: Nightshade and Illness*.

The GI tract of some people with rheumatoid arthritis may be more permeable than normal. NSAIDs may make the abnormality worse, because of its tendency to promote ulcers and bleeding in the GI tract, as discussed in Chapter 2. Researchers agree that diet may alter the immune or inflammatory responses, or that specific foods may act as antigens in hypersensitive people, triggering rheumatic symptoms. And the permeability of the GI tract "opens the door" for protein fragments to enter the body and provoke an inflammatory, autoimmune response. At least one well-known physician believes that increased gut permeability is itself due to inflammation of the intestinal wall caused by exposure to dairy and other animal products, which leads to more antigens entering the body. Unfortunately, none of this "proves" the link between certain foods and rheumatoid arthritis.

One consistent finding is that fasting has been found to improve the symptoms in rheumatoid arthritis. In some cases, water fasts of up to a week or even 10 days have been used, relieving symptoms such as pain and stiffness, but these symptoms return when the patients resume normal eating. Such fasts are extremely dangerous and should be avoided unless supervised by a qualified physician. Also, some patients improve on experimental diets involving lab-produced "elemental" diets, but also usually experience a return of symptoms when they resume normal eating.

Most experts agree that, although rare, some rheumatoid arthritis patients do have clinical symptoms associated with food sensitivity. In one recent study, 30% of rheumatoid arthritis patients claimed to have food sensitive or "allergic" arthritis, and careful testing confirmed definite sensitivity in 3 of the 16 patients. In another somewhat larger study, 12 of 27 rheumatoid arthritis patients randomly assigned to a group eating a vegan, gluten-free diet showed marked reduction in symptoms. If representative, these preliminary studies indicate that somewhere between 6% and 45% of rheumatoid arthritis cases are definitely linked to diet: foods consumed trigger the inflammation, swelling, and other symptoms associated with rheumatoid arthritis.

These results have led some researchers to think that changing to a high-fiber, low-animal-product diet might beneficially change bacteria in the gut, in particular reducing the population of a common bug, *proteus mirabilis*, as all those who benefited from the diet showed this change. In yet another study, the vegan diet produced different microflora in the gut between those who benefited from the diet and those who did not, although the specific bacterial changes were not identified. Keep in mind that diets in general, such as vegan or elimination, may be only rarely beneficial and that no dietary manipulations have been beneficial for everyone. Such statements are of course meaningless to you if you happen to be one of those who have benefited. You have, in effect, found a cure for the incurable!

The Vegan Diet Option

There is one type of therapeutic diet, however, that is not hard to follow and has been shown to benefit a small but definite group with rheumatoid arthritis who do have allergic reactions to animal products: the vegan diet.

If you have rheumatoid arthritis, try the vegan diet by all means. I'll show you how to do it safely, and if you don't see any obvious benefits after two or three months, then return to the basic diet as outlined in Chapter 8. Keep in mind that the vegan diet is a radical change: You will have to eliminate almost all common foods, processed foods, restaurant foods, and so on. You eat essentially only home-prepared fruit, vegetable, and grain meals with no meat, dairy, or additives such as preservatives, flavorings or colorings, or alcohol. Dinner parties, snacks at ball games, and eating on the go are difficult if not impossible when you follow this diet, but if normal eating habits are causing the symptoms of rheumatoid arthritis, then you perhaps have more to gain than to lose.

Vegan Diet Tips

Nutritionally, the carbohydrate and fat content of a vegan diet is easy: the same whole grains, fruits, and vegetables providing carbohydrates for a nonvegetarian diet also work here. The recommended oils — olive and canola for cooking, with enough flaxseed oil on salads to provide needed essential fatty acids — also work here. You never have to worry about getting too much saturated fat, because there isn't any. Protein intake for most people, as I discussed in Chapter 8, is usually at least double our requirements in America, and meeting the recommended 15% of total calories is pretty easy. Soy-based products, including "fake" meats, tofu, and tempeh, as well as dried peas, beans, and lentils, are all excellent sources. Rice- and soy-milk products are now widely distributed through supermarkets, as are many fake meat products, from "bacon" to "chopped hamburger." Since individual calorie requirements vary quite a bit, an easier way to determine your protein requirements is to multiply your weight by a factor related to your lifestyle. We have provided a table with this calculation for you to refer to (see p. 210), and this method usually agrees well with the 15% of total required calories recommended by the USDA.

Many experts have noted over the years that a vegan diet is often deficient in certain vitamins and minerals, and it is true that great care is needed to make a vegan diet truly complete. However, it is simple to supplement your diet with the basic multivitamin/mineral supplement, with added B, C, E, and calcium/magnesium as described in Chapter 8; then all requirements will have been met. The basic supplement provides the missing vitamins D, B-2, and B-12, as well as calcium, selenium, iron, and zinc. Additionally, some common foods suitable for vegans, such as breads, cereals, and soy/sesame milk, are often fortified with vitamins and minerals, too. Nutrition experts also counsel in favor of supplementing the essential fatty acid content of a strict diet with foods rich in alpha linolenic acid (ALA), such as flaxseed oil, dark green leafy vegetables, pumpkin seeds, walnuts, and several beans, including soy, kidney, lima, navy, and great northern.

Following are some specific guidelines for creating a healthy vegan menu. See the Resources section for some recommended cookbooks.

• Eat 6-11 servings per day of whole-grain products, fortified if available.

• Eat 3-5 servings of vegetables: raw, steamed, or stir-fried.

• Eat 2-4 servings of fruits.

• Eat 4-8 protein servings (an average adult woman needs 60 grams; an average adult male, 70 grams).

• Learn how to combine protein sources for higher protein utilization, for instance, grains with beans, or legumes (dried peas, beans, and lentils) with seeds (sesame, pumpkin, sun-flower, etc.).

• Use oils and high-fat foods (nuts, avocados, seeds, even some granolas) sparingly.

• Use highly sweetened and very salty foods sparingly.

• Take a good multivitamin/mineral supplement, with added Vitamins C, E, and calcium/magnesium.

• Watch your weight; if it drops too low, add more high-calorie foods (nuts, seeds, etc.).

• If you do not see any improvement in rheumatic symptoms after several weeks, try also eliminating high-gluten products such as wheat and corn.

• If eliminating wheat and corn helps, there are many resources available: check your library, health food store, and bookstore for gluten-free recipes and information.

• If your symptoms respond to a vegan diet, you may add back foods one by one, and eliminate any that cause a return of symptoms. Some experts recommend challenging your body twice with a suspect food to make sure it really does trigger symptoms. It makes sense to add fat-free dairy first, because these foods are highly nutritious, and, in at least one study, rheumatoid arthritis symptoms did not return when dairy products were returned to the diet.

• If there is still no improvement after four to six weeks, feel free to resume normal eating.

Protein Sources Table

PROTEIN FOOD	Serving Size	Calories	Protein Grams	Calories per Gram
Dried beans, peas, lentils cooked	1/2 cup	100	7	14
Tofu	3 oz	75	7.5	10
Tempeh	4 oz	200	20	10
Veggie hot dog	1 wiener	55	11	5
Veggie deli slices	4 slices	70	15	5
Veggie burger	2 oz pattie	98	8	12
Soy milk	1 cup	115	8	14

Note: rice milk contains only 1 gram of protein per cup; not a good alternative protein source.

Protein Requirements Table

To use the following table, find your weight in pounds in the left-hand column, and read across to find your protein needs, in grams, in the column that best describes your activity level.

Protein Requirements Table

Weight (in lbs)	Activity Level		
	Low	Moderate	High
100	40	50	75
110	44	55	83
120	48	60	90
130	52	65	98
140	56	70	105
150	60	75	113
160	64	80	120
170	68	85	128
180	72	90	135
190	76	95	143
200	80	100	150
210	84	105	158
220	88	110	165
230	92	115	173
240	96	120	180
250	100	125	188

Protein requirements vary according to age and activity level as follows:

LOW – for most adults who are sedentary to moderately active.

MODERATE – for active adults who regularly (daily) engage in fast-paced sports or other athletic training, or heavy manual labor, such as lifting, shoveling, etc.

HIGH – for a growing athlete, or an adult who is using weight training to build muscle mass.

Resources

Following is a general guide to some books, periodicals, and websites that may be helpful to supplement your knowledge about arthritis, weight loss, exercise, alternative therapies, and nutrition. (Because the content of the World Wide Web changes constantly, use search engines to find the most comprehensive and current list of helpful sites.)

General Resources for Arthritis, including Current Medical News and Information about Traditional and Alternative Therapies

The Arthritis Foundation:
1330 W. Peachtree St.
Atlanta, GA 30309
(404) 872-7100

www.arthritis.org – "Arthritis Today" magazine; common questions; free brochures; books and other products; message boards; how to find local chapters; position statement about MSM; etc.

The Arthritis Foundation's Guide to Alternative Remedies, by Judith Horstman (Arthritis Foundation, 1999)

arthritis.about.com/health/arthritis

pslgroup.com/arthritis.htm – latest research, medical news, fact sheets, discussion groups, list of related sites

rheumatology.org – American College of Rheumatology

nutriteam.com/coburn.htm – manufacturer's website; includes James Coburn's testimonial

lifetel.com/msm/missinglink.htm

Vegan / Vegetarian Diet

vegsource.org

vegan.com

vrg.org (Vegetarian Resource Group)

eatright.org/adap1197.html (American Dietetic Association Position Statement on Vegetarian Diets)

DrMcdougall.com (Dr. John McDougall's general health newsletter; medical updates and vegan recipes)

Simply Vegan, by Debra Wasserman (3rd ed.; Baltimore, MD: Vegetarian Resource Group, 1999).

Eco-Cuisine: An Ecological Approach to Gourmet Vegetarian Cooking, by Ron Pickarski (Berkeley, CA: Ten Speed Press, 1995)

How it all Vegan, by Tanya Barnard and Sarah Kramer (Vancouver, BC: Arsenal Pulp Press, 1999).

The Vegetarian Way, Virginia Messina, MPH, RD, and Mark Messina, PhD (New York: Crown Publishing Group, 1996)

Becoming Vegetarian: The Complete Guide to Adopting a Vegetarian Diet, by Vesanto Melina, Brenda Davis, and Victoria Harrison (Summertown, TN: The Book Publishing Co., 1995)

The Dietician's Guide to Vegetarian Diets: Issues and Applications, by Virginia Messina, MPH, RD, and Mark Messina, PhD (a textbook)

The Vegan Handbook, by Debra Wasserman and Reed Margels, PhD, RD (Baltimore, MD: Vegetarian Resource Group, 1996)

The Vegetarian Times Vegetarian Beginner's Guide (IDG Books Worldwide, 1996). Also see, by the same authors, *The Vegetarian Times Low-Fat and Fast* (series), and *The Vegetarian Times Complete Cookbook.*

Vegetarian Cooking for Everyone, by Deborah Madison (Broadway Books, 1997)

The Complete Vegetarian Cuisine (rev. ed.), by Rose Elliott (Pantheon Books, 1997)

"The Vegetarian Times" (www.vegetariantimes.com) or call 977-717-8923 to subscribe

"The Vegetarian Journal" (available from the Vegetarian Resource Group, PO Box 1463, Baltimore, MD, 21203; 410-366-8343)

General Nutrition

Nancy Clark's Sports Nutrition Guidebook, 2nd ed., by Nancy Clark (Champaign, IL: Human Kinetics, 1996).

The Nutrition Doctor's A-to-Z Food Counter, by Dr. Ed Blonz (New York: Penguin, 1999).

Prevention Magazine's Nutrition Advisor, by Mark Bricklin (Emmaus, PA: Rodale Press, 1993).

"Nutrition Action" (newsletter of the Center for Science in the Public Interest, 1875 Connecticut Ave, NW, #300, Washington, DC 20009-5729). Up-to-date information for consumers about food safety, nutrition research, healthy eating suggestions, and so on.

Weight Management

In addition to basic information about healthy weight management, many of the following sites offer interactive tools such as individual diet planners, menu ideas, and food analysis; a chance to ask experts questions about dieting and nutrition; support chat rooms; and other features.

Cyberdiet.com

Intelihealth.com

Nourishnet.com

Obesity.com

Prevention.com

YourBetterHealth.com

Registered Dieticians

For individualized advice about diet, we recommend consulting a registered dietician (RD). These health professionals have fulfilled specific educational requirements, have passed a registration exam, and are a recognized member of the nation's largest organization of nutrition professionals, The American Dietetic Association. Contact them for a referral to a professional in your area.

> **American Dietetic Association**
> 216 W. Jackson Blvd.
> Chicago, IL 60606-6995
> Tel: (312) 899-0040 x4750
> Fax: (312) 899-4739
> website: www.eatright.org

800-366-1655 (toll-free) for recorded messages about current nutrition topics and to get a referral to a registered dietician in your local area.

900-225-5267 for individualized answers to your questions from a registered dietician. Charges: $1.95 first minute, $.95 each additional minute, average call four minutes.

Books on Walking, Swimming, and Cycling

Walking Medicine, by Gary Yanker (McGraw-Hill, 1992)

Walk Aerobics, by Les Snowdon (Overlook Press, 1995)

WALKFIT for a Better Body, by Kathy Smith (Warner Books, 1994)

Fitness Cycling, by Chris Carmichael and Edmund R. Burke (Human Kinetics, 1994)

Power Pacing for Indoor Cycling, by Kristopher Kory and Thomas Seabourne (Human Kinetics, 1999)

Cycling Past 50, by Joe Friel (Human Kinetics, 1998)

All-American Aquatic Handbook, by Jane Katz (Allyn & Bacon, 1996)

Swimming for Total Fitness, by Jane Katz (Main Street Books, rev. ed. 1993)

Complete Book of Swimming, by Dr. Phillip Whitten (Random House, 1994)

Resources from The American Yoga Association

For free information about Yoga, including a complete catalog, visit our website, or send a self-addressed envelope stamped with postage for two ounces to the following address:

> **American Yoga Association**
> P.O. Box 19986
> Sarasota, FL 34276

If you have a specific question about Yoga and would like a personal reply, write to the address above, or contact us by telephone, fax, or E-mail:

> Telephone (941) 927-4977
> Fax: (941) 921-9844
> E-mail: info@americanyogaassociation.org
> Website: www.americanyogaassociation.org

We offer classes in the Cleveland, Ohio, area. For more information, write or call:

American Yoga Association
P.O. Box 18105
Cleveland Hts, OH 44106
Telephone (216) 556-1313

Books

The American Yoga Association Beginner's Manual (Simon & Schuster, 1987). Complete instructions for over 90 Yoga exercises and breathing techniques; three 10-week curriculum outlines, and chapters on nutrition, philosophy, stress management, nutrition, pregnancy, and more.

The American Yoga Association's New Yoga Challenge (NTC/Contemporary, 1997). Routines for Energy, Strength, Flexibility, Focus, and Stability offer more vigorous Yoga workouts for body and mind. The last chapter, "The Powerful Individual," teaches you how to design your own routine.

The American Yoga Association Wellness Book (Kensington, 1996). A basic routine to maintain health and well-being, plus chapters on how Yoga can specifically help with arthritis, heart disease, back pain, PMS & menopause, weight management, insomnia, headaches, and eight other health conditions.

The American Yoga Association's Yoga for Sports (NTC/Contemporary Books, 2000). A comprehensive book for every athlete, including techniques for bringing the physical and emotional bodies together to attain peak performance. Includes a core routine of exercise, breathing, and meditation, plus specific exercise routines for dozens of individual sports, team sports, and coaches.

Conversations with Swami Lakshmanjoo, Volume I: Aspects of Kashmir Shaivism (American Yoga Association, 1995). Edited transcripts of Alice Christensen's interviews with Swami Lakshmanjoo, talking about his childhood and early years in Yoga, plus some basic concepts in the philosophy of Kashmir Shaivism.

Conversations with Swami Lakshmanjoo, Volume II: The Yamas and Niyamas of Patanjali (American Yoga Association, 1998). Edited transcripts of Alice Christensen's dialogues with Swami Lakshmanjoo about these essential ethical guidelines in Yoga.

Easy Does It Yoga (Fireside/Simon & Schuster, 1999). For those with physical limitations, this book includes instruction in specially adapted Yoga exercises that can be done in a chair or in bed, breathing techniques, and meditation.

The Easy Does It Yoga Trainer's Guide (Kendall-Hunt, 1995). A complete manual for how to begin teaching the Easy Does It Yoga program to adults with physical limitations due to age, convalescence, substance abuse, injury, or obesity. Excellent for health professionals, activities directors, physical therapists, home health aides, and others who work with the elderly or in rehabilitative services.

Heart Health: An American Yoga Association Wellness Guide (Kensington Publishing, 2001). A complete program for preventing or reversing heart disease, including a unique routine of Yoga exercise, breathing, and meditation training, plus instruction in self-directed fantasy techniques, a special walking program, a section on stress management, and a comprehensive heart-healthy diet and nutrition program.

The Light of Yoga (American Yoga Association, 1997). A chronicle of the unusual circumstances that catapulted Alice Christensen into Yoga practice in the early 1950s, including the teachers and experiences that shaped her first years of study.

Meditation (American Yoga Association, 1994). A collection of excerpts from lectures and classes on the subject of meditation, including a section of questions and answers from students.

20-Minute Yoga Workouts (Ballantine, 1995). Brief routines that anyone can fit into the busiest schedule. Includes chapters on women's issues (including pregnancy), toning and shaping, the "20-minute challenge," and workouts to do when you're away from home.

Reflections of Love (American Yoga Association, 1994). A collection of excerpts from Alice Christensen's lectures and classes on the subject of love.

Weight Management: An American Yoga Association Wellness Guide (Kensington Publishing, 2001). A complete program for weight management in six parts: Yoga exercise, breathing, and meditation, combined with fantasy techniques, a special walking program, and a healthy and enjoyable diet plan.

Yoga of the Heart: Ten Ethical Principles for Gaining Limitless Growth, Confidence, and Achievement (Daybreak/Rodale Books, 1998). A clear, direct presentation of ten essential ethics — Nonviolence, Truthfulness, Nonstealing, Celibacy, Nonhoarding, Purity, Contentment, Tolerance, Study, and Remembrance — that help a person realize the power and support of joining the physical and spiritual bodies. Each chapter includes suggestions for how to start practicing, common pitfalls along the way, and many examples from students' experiences and mythology to illustrate the journey.

Audiotapes

Complete Relaxation and Meditation with Alice Christensen. A two-tape audiocassette program that features three guided meditation sessions of varying lengths, including instruction in a seated posture, plus a discussion of meditation experiences.

The "I Love You" Meditation Technique. This technique begins with the experience of a more conscious connection with the breath through love. It then extends this feeling throughout the body and mind in relaxation and meditation. This tape teaches you the beauty of loving yourself and it removes unseen fear.

Videotapes

Basic Yoga. A complete introduction to Yoga that includes exercise, breathing, and relaxation and meditation techniques. Provides detailed instruction in all the techniques including variations for more or less flexibility, plus a special limbering routine and back-strengthening exercises. Features a 30-minute daily routine demonstrated in the setting of a Yoga class.

Conversations with Swami Lakshmanjoo. A set of three videotapes in which Alice Christensen introduces Swami Lakshmanjoo and talks with him about his background, the philosophy of Kashmir Shaivism, and other topics in Yoga. (Some material corresponds to Volume I of the book *Aspects of Kashmir Shaivism* described above.)

Videotape Lecture Series

These are videotaped classes of Alice Christensen, filmed in a casual setting in a lecture/discussion format with a small group of students.

Ethics in Yoga (25 tapes): An in-depth examination of ten ethical guidelines from Classical Yoga philosophy (Nonviolence, Truth, Nonstealing, Nonhoarding, Celibacy, Purity, Contentment, Study, Tolerance, and Remembrance), also incorporating portions of my videotaped conversations with the great Yoga master Lakshmanjoo of Kashmir.

The Hero in Yoga (27 tapes): Using as a text Joseph Campbell's landmark work *The Hero with a Thousand Faces*, this series correlates the hero's journey with modern Americans' personal search for meaning and self-knowledge in life.

How to Choose a Qualified Yoga Teacher

So far, no national or international certification program for yoga teachers exists, and it is unlikely that it will, because of the traditional nature of Yoga instruction. For many thousands of years, Yoga was transmitted from teacher to student on a one-to-one basis; only comparatively recently has Yoga been offered in a group class format. Advanced practice of Yoga still is best undertaken on a one-to-one basis, if you are lucky enough to find a competent teacher who is willing to teach you. In my opinion, teaching Yoga should not be viewed as a hobby or a sideline undertaken by someone who reads a couple of books and decides to become a Yoga teacher; he or she must be under the constant supervision of his or her personal Yoga teacher. This relationship between teacher and student is taken very seriously by both parties and is never entered into lightly.

People are constantly asking us to recommend teachers in their area. Because of my belief in the strict training required for the teaching of Yoga, I have made it a policy never to recommend a teacher unless I have trained the person. I cannot take responsibility for other people's teaching. This does not mean that there are no competent teachers available; you may just have to search a little harder. If you are not sure where to start looking, inquire about adult education programs at local schools; look for flyers posted ·in local health food stores and bookstores or notices in community papers; and inquire at dance and massage studios.

In the following paragraphs, I have outlined what I believe are the minimum requirements for a competent teacher of Yoga.

1. Daily practice of Yoga exercise, breathing, and meditation. No one can make progress in Yoga without a serious commitment to daily practice. A teacher must have this support in order to build the solid foundation of experience that is required before he or she can show others how to achieve that experience; daily practice is also needed to maintain the strength and health necessary for the extra demands of teaching.

2. Regular contact with a teacher. No teacher can work effectively in a vacuum, and no one becomes so advanced that he or she does not need the guidance and support of his or her own teacher.

3. Study of the important Yoga texts. Study is one of the five observances that are part of the essential eight "limbs" of Yoga practice (see #4, below). A teacher needs to have an intensive background of study that includes

Patanjali's *Yoga Sutras*, the *Hatha Yoga Pradipika*, the *Bhagavad Gita*, and all world philosophies, at the very least.

4. Ethical behavior. The five *yamas* (meaning "restraints": Nonviolence, Truthfulness, Nonstealing, periods of Celibacy, Nonhoarding) and the five *niyamas* (meaning "observances": Purity, Contentment, Tolerance, Study, Remembrance) are the first two limbs in Patanjali's system of classical Yoga (called "Ashtanga Yoga"). The remaining six limbs are 1) physical exercises *(asana)*, 2) breathing techniques *(pranayama)*, 3) withdrawal of the mind from the senses *(pratyahara)*, 4) concentration, defined as selective and voluntary dishabituation *(dharana)*, 5) meditation *(dhyana)*, and 6) absorption, or ultimate union with the self *(samadhi)*. My teacher Lakshmanjoo once said that, like a child developing in the womb whose limbs grow all at once, rather than one by one, these eight limbs must be developed simultaneously.

The ethical guidelines of the yamas and niyamas are a part of Yoga practice not for moralistic reasons but because they support and protect the student during the unfolding of personal experience in meditation. A teacher needs this support and protection for the same reasons as well as to help reduce the interference of personal ego in the teaching process.

An ethical Yoga teacher conducts classes in a responsible, safe, and aware manner; organizes classes that are not too large for each student to receive individual attention; and never pushes students beyond their limitations. Sexual involvement with students is absolutely prohibited.

5. A healthy vegetarian diet. Although you do not need to be a vegetarian to practice Yoga, a Yoga teacher must conform to different standards. Someone who is taking responsibility for teaching others how to use Yoga meditation techniques must have the steadiness and nonviolent attitude that can only be attained through a vegetarian diet. It goes without saying that a teacher should not smoke or use drugs (other than prescription medication) or misuse alcohol.

6. Training in basic anatomy and the effects of Yoga techniques. A teacher must be able to vary the techniques according to each student's ability and know how to advise students with common medical conditions such as hypertension, arthritis, and back problems. I also believe that a teacher should be able to recognize when a student needs professional psychological counseling and be familiar with community services to which to refer the student.

7. Ability to separate Yoga from religion. I have seen many poor-quality instructors take on the trappings and robes of Hinduism or some other religion to give themselves an authority through packaging rather than through the authenticity of their own Yoga practice. This practice severely misrepresents Yoga. Yoga is not a religion; it predates Hinduism — as well as all known religious practices — and its techniques have been used throughout the world. Yoga is a system of nonreligious, transcultural techniques that can develop greater self-knowledge and awareness. Unlike a religion, Yoga does not require adherence to certain creeds or beliefs, nor does it require obeisance to any particular prophet or god. Yoga is not ritualistic, nor is it occult. The texts of Yoga are not scriptures but rather handbooks or guidelines of how to use the techniques safely and what kinds of experiences might be possible. Everyone has a right to their personal religious beliefs, but a teacher must never impose his or her personal beliefs on students in a Yoga class.

About The American Yoga Association

The American Yoga Association teaches a comprehensive and balanced program of Yoga that includes the Hatha Yoga exercises and breathing techniques as well as meditation. Rather than stressing physical culture for its own sake, our core curriculum acknowledges the deeper possibilities of Yoga by teaching meditation and by encouraging the inner-directed awareness that eventually leads to greater self-knowledge. This reliance on individual experience and feeling is a central theme in the science of Yoga, and it underlies the philosophical system of Kashmir Shaivism which supports our line of teaching. Our goal is to offer the highest quality Yoga instruction possible. There are two American Yoga Association Centers in the United States.

About the Author

Alice Christensen stands out as a Yoga teacher with the rare ability to make the often-complex ideas and techniques of Yoga accessible to our Western outlook and lifestyle. She established the American Yoga Association in 1968, the first nonprofit organization in the United States dedicated to education in Yoga.

She has consistently presented Yoga in a clear, classical manner for over forty years. She presents Yoga without dogma or prescription, as a potent avenue for individual inquiry. She has designed programs of Yoga that can be used to enhance any lifestyle. Whether the goal is to maintain health or to explore the nature of the self, her programs can be used to achieve a wide range of goals.

Index

208-209
Vegetarianism, 162, 180, 190
Vioxx, 23, 33
Virus, 24
Vitamin A, 180, 182, 185
Vitamin B-complex, 52, 69, 160, 180,
    194-196, 208
    as alternative therapy, 190, 194-195
    and SAM-e, 202
Vitamin B-1, 195
Vitamin B-12, 180, 185, 195, 208
Vitamin B-2, 180, 195, 208
Vitamin B-3, 194, 195
Vitamin B-5, 194, 195, 196
Vitamin B-6, 195, 196
Vitamin C, 52, 152, 157, 158 ,178, 180,
    182, 185, 187, 188, 208, 209
Vitamin D, 157, 179, 180, 183, 185
Vitamin E, 25, 152, 157, 158, 178, 180,
    182, 184, 185, 188, 208, 209
Vitamin brands, 186
Vitamins, 178-188 (*also see* specific
    vitamins)
Voltaren, 32
Walking contemplation, 139-151
Walking,
    hints for, 147
    schedule for, 144-145
Warm-up for exercise session, 145-146
Warm-ups (Yoga), 51, 53-79
Water, 94
"Wear and tear," 1, 17
Weight,
    arthritis and, 2, 20-21
    depression and, 153
    exercise and, 29
    self-esteem and, 153
Weight loss, 27
    activity and, 156-157
    diet and, 38
    stress of, 36
    tips for, 154-157
Wheat and corn, 209 (*also see* Gluten)
Whirlwind, 87-89

Wind sprints, 149
Women, supplements and, 179
Wrist tape technique, 41-43, 154-155
Yoga breathing, how it works, 36
Yoga exercise,
    alcohol and, 12
    benefits of, 36
    breathing and, 48-49
    caffeine and, 12
    clothing, equipment, environment
        for, 11-12
    daily practice of, 50-51
    ethics and, 38-41
    food and, 12
    goals for, 9-10
    modifying, 9
    meaning of word, 6
    medication and, 12
    menstrual cycle and, 13
    nursing and, 13
    osteoarthritis and, 30
    pacing, 49-50
    pregnancy and, 13
    range-of-motion in, 10
    rheumatoid arthritis and, 26
    scheduling, 10, 11, 12, 43-44
Yoga teacher, 13
Zinc, 180, 181, 185, 208